Case Studies in LPN/LVN Nursing

Janis McMillan PhD, MSN, RN, CNE

Clinical Professor
College of Nursing
Northern Arizona University
Flagstaff, Arizona

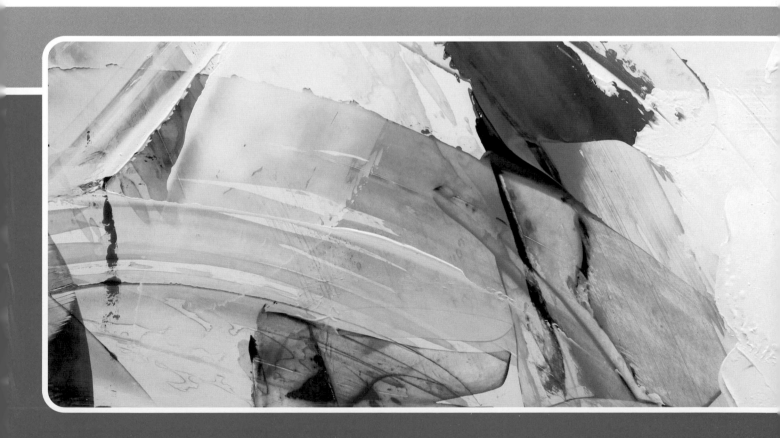

ELSEVIER

Elsevier
3251 Riverport Lane
St. Louis, Missouri 63043

Notice

Practitioners and researchers must always rely on their own experience and knowledge in evaluating and using any information, methods, compounds or experiments described herein. Because of rapid advances in the medical sciences, in particular, independent verification of diagnoses and drug dosages should be made. To the fullest extent of the law, no responsibility is assumed by Elsevier, authors, editors or contributors for any injury and/or damage to persons or property as a matter of products liability, negligence or otherwise, or from any use or operation of any methods, products, instructions, or ideas contained in the material herein.

Senior Content Strategist: Brandi Graham
Director, Content Development: Ellen Wurm-Cutter
Sr. Content Development Manager: Somodatta Roy Choudhury
Publishing Services Manager: Deepthi Unni
Project Manager: Thoufiq Mohammed
Design Direction: Amy Buxton

Printed in India

Last digit is the print number: 9 8 7 6 5 4 3 2 1

Working together
to grow libraries in
developing countries

www.elsevier.com • www.bookaid.org

*To my family, who have always been my biggest cheerleaders and
who always support me, I love you.
To the nurses I have worked with over my 40-year career in so many settings,
units, and hospitals, your love and care for countless patients and clients,
and for me, has inspired me to be my best.
To my teaching colleagues, who inspire me with their dedication
to teaching excellence.*

Contributors

Heather Holland Ashby, MSN, RNC-OB, CNE
Associate Clinical Professor
College of Nursing
Northern Arizona University
Flagstaff, Arizona
Chapter 22: Prenatal Care
Chapter 23: Labor
Chapter 24: Assessment of Newborn
Chapter 25: Preterm Infant
Chapter 26: Postpartum/Mood Disorder
Chapter 27: Respiratory Syncytial Virus (RSV)
Chapter 34: Pediatric Asthma

Garrett S. Mitchell, MSN, RN, CMSRN, CNOR
Assistant Clinical Professor
College of Nursing
Northern Arizona University
Flagstaff, Arizona
Chapter 7: Unfolding Case Study of the Perioperative Process
Chapter 16: DVT/PE
Chapter 32: Pediatric Fracture

The National Council of State Boards of Nursing (NCSBN) has begun testing nursing candidates using the Next-Generation NCLEX® (NGN) Examination for nursing licensure. The NGN includes traditional NCLEX questions and has added new test items to measure clinical judgment to support client safety. The nurse uses clinical judgment to make decisions in client care and uses nursing knowledge to observe, gather information, prioritize the information, generate evidence-based solutions in planning care, deliver safe care, and evaluate the outcomes of that care. Per the NCSBN 2023 PN Test plan, clinical judgment content may be tested using a case study or individual standalone questions.

This workbook is designed for students enrolled in prelicensure programs in preparation for practical nursing (PN) practice and consists of unfolding case study questions. **Answer keys** are available to instructors only through the accompanying Evolve companion website at evolve.elsevier.com.

- These unfolding case studies will assist you to develop clinical reasoning and clinical judgment as they better reflect real-world nursing care.
- Developing clinical judgment is crucial to safe patient care in whatever settings you practice during your nursing career.
- Practicing NGN unfolding case studies will prepare you for success on the Next-Generation NCLEX® Examination (NGN) and is intended for use throughout your nursing program. Case studies are available for basic foundational care through specialty practice and demonstrate multiple NGN-style test items.

A case study contains six items that are associated with the same client presentation and share unfolding client information. Each case study will test all six of the following clinical skills:

- Recognize Cues: Filtering information from different sources (e.g., signs, symptoms, medical history)—this is "what matters the most?"
- Analyze Cues: Linking the recognized cues to the client's clinical presentation and establishing probable client needs, concerns, or problems—this is the "what could it mean?"
- Prioritize Hypothesis: Evaluating and ranking hypotheses according to priority (urgency, likelihood, risk, difficulty, time, etc.)—this is "where do I start?"
- Generate Solutions: Identifying expected outcomes and using hypotheses to define a set of interventions for the expected outcome—this is "what can I do?"
- Take Action: Implementing the solution(s) that addresses the highest priorities; sometimes no action is an action itself—this is "what will I do?"
- Evaluate Outcomes: Comparing observed outcomes against expected outcomes—this is "did it help?"

The NGN exam includes a new case study-based format and many new question types. The new NGN formatted questions include the following:

- Highlight: These items include reading from the client's chart and then highlighting words or phrases in a paragraph or table that answers the question.
- Drag and drop: These questions ask you to move or place options into answer spaces; you may need to number items in order or check off items that answer the question.
- Drop down: These items can have two or more parts; you will select the missing word or phrase option from a list; these options will complete a sentence, sentences, or a table.
- Matrix/grid: These items are multiple-choice or multiple-response items that are in a matrix or grid; you will select one or more answer options for each row or column.
- Extended multiple response: These are very much like the current "select all that apply" questions but may have up to 10 options to choose from; there is also a "select N" that tells you the correct number of items that you need to choose (i.e., "choose the four findings . . .") and the formatting may look like an order set where you will select one or more options from multiple categories.

Acknowledgment

My sincere appreciation goes out to the many individuals who assisted my efforts in writing this workbook.

I would like to acknowledge and thank all of the staff at Elsevier for their tremendous assistance: holding my hand, answering question upon question, and providing support throughout the preparation and production of this publication. Thanks to all of you.

I could not have done this without the collaboration with my two contributing authors, Heather Ashby (OB and pediatrics) and Garrett Mitchell (fundamentals and medical-surgical), who laughed and learned with me and contributed excellent case studies related to their areas of expertise. You are amazing and I'm so blessed to call you friends and colleagues.

Lastly, I extend a thank you to all of my nursing students, past, present, and future. You are why I do what I do. Your enthusiasm renews me and continuously shapes my own teaching and learning. You remind me of how important the art and science of nursing are, of the incredible value of evidence-based practice, and of the joy of making a difference in someone's life. You allow me to touch so many people through you when I'm not even present. I'm so proud of you!

Contents

Section 4: Pediatrics

Section 5: Mental Health

Section 6: Geriatrics

Section 7: Leadership Management

Infection Control

Outcome

The learner will correctly identify required actions to manage a client with infection control needs.

Scenario

A 48-year-old client with a history of diabetes mellitus and obesity stepped on a piece of glass while walking barefoot in a park several days ago. The LVN has a practical nursing student working with them for this shift. They are standing at the client's bedside after the patient arrives in the unit.

Health History	Nurses' Notes	**Healthcare Provider Orders**	Laboratory Results

1040:
- Admit to medical floor, diagnosis cellulitis left foot
- Wound culture and sensitivity
- Tetanus booster IM
- Daily dressing change left foot

Health History	**Nurses' Notes**	Healthcare Provider Orders	Laboratory Results

Vital Signs	1135
Temperature (F/C)	100.9°/38.2°
Heart Rate (bpm)	94
Respirations (bpm)	20
Blood Pressure (mmHg)	128/72

Nurses' Notes

1135: Admitted client to two-bed room. Settled in bed, oriented to room. Client is crying. The client states recently divorced, is all alone, and is really scared. Wound on the bottom of the left foot is red, open, and draining a yellow-green discharge. Redness around the wound is 7 cm × 5 cm × 9 cm, area marked.

1. NGN Item Type: Highlight Text

1.1.1 Highlight the assessment findings that require follow-up by the LVN and nursing student.

Health History	Nurses' Notes	**Healthcare Provider Orders**	Laboratory Results

1040:
- Admit to medical floor, diagnosis cellulitis left foot
- Wound culture and sensitivity
- Tetanus booster IM
- Daily dressing change left foot

Health History	Nurses' Notes	Healthcare Provider Orders	Laboratory Results

Vital Signs	1135
Temperature (F/C)	100.9°/38.2°
Heart Rate (bpm)	94
Respirations (bpm)	20
Blood Pressure (mmHg)	128/72

Nurses' Notes

1135: Admitted client to two-bed room. Settled in bed, oriented to room. Client is crying. The client states recently divorced, is all alone, and is really scared. Wound on the bottom of the left foot is red, open, and draining a yellow-green discharge. Redness around the wound is 7 cm × 5 cm × 9 cm, area marked.

2. NGN Item Type: Multiple Response Select All That Apply

1.1.2 The LVN asks the practical nursing student to identify which of the nursing assessment findings support the use of standard precautions for this client. Select all that apply.

A. T 100.9°F (38.2°C)
B. Wound is red and open
C. Wound is draining a yellow-green discharge
D. Tetanus booster IM
E. Standing at the bedside to ask client questions
F. Dressing change daily
G. Documenting nurses' notes and vital signs in the computer
H. Taking the client's pulse

Scenario

Two hours later after documenting the client's current status, the LVN and the student discuss the potential treatment plan.

Health History	Nurses' Notes	Healthcare Provider Orders	Laboratory Results

1330:
Vancomycin order received; vancomycin IV hung by RN. Client placed in precautions for possible MRSA in the wound. Rapid MRSA test sent to the lab.

1. NGN Item Type: Drop-Down Cloze

1.2.1 Choose the *most likely* options for the information missing from the statements below by selecting from the lists of options provided.

Based on the patient's condition, the practical nursing student states the client's **priority** need will be to prevent _____1_____ and anticipates the client will be placed in _____2_____ precautions.

Options for 1	Options for 2
Sepsis	Airborne
Loneliness	Contact
Hyperthermia	Droplet

2. NGN Item Type: Matrix Multiple Choice

1.2.2 **The LVN asks the practical nursing student to consider precautionary measures for the client. Use an X to identify the indicated or contraindicated nursing interventions for this client. Each row must only have one response option selected.**

Nursing Interventions	Indicated	Contraindicated
Save gloves to wear later in care of the client if not visibly soiled		
Wear respiratory device (N95 respirator)		
Place client in a private room		
Wear glove for contact with blood or body fluids		
Wash hands after touching blood and body fluids or removing gloves		
Place patient in a room with negative air pressure		
Wear PPE gown when changing the client's dressing		
Place mask on client when client needs to leave the room		
Use soap and water to wash hands every time and not alcohol-based hand rub		
When wearing a gown, remove it before taking off gloves		
Wear goggles or face shield when changing the wound dressing if drainage might splatter		

Scenario

The client is placed in isolation. Several hours later, the rapid MRSA test returns positive for MRSA in the left foot wound. The client's sister and family arrive and are encouraged to stay and visit the client. The client has a lot of questions and states, "I've never known anyone who has had to do this before." The LVN asks the nursing student what she would include when reinforcing teaching with this client.

1. NGN Item Type: Multiple Response Select All That Apply

1.3.1 **When reinforcing teaching to the client and their family, the practical nursing student includes which of the following information? Select all that apply.**
   A. You have MRSA in your wound, which is easily transmitted by direct patient contact or contact with items in the patient's room.
   B. Good nutrition and more than adequate fluid intake will be important for your healing.
   C. Your family does not need to wear a mask while they are in the room as long as they stay at least 3 feet away from the client.
   D. Let me show you the specifics on how to wash your hands with soap and water or use the alcohol-based hand rub.
   E. You will need to stay in your room the whole time you are in isolation, you won't be able to leave it.
   F. There will be a sign on the door to remind staff and visitors of what to do with this type of isolation.

Scenario

The next day, the practical nursing student enters the client's room and puts on their gloves and then their gown. The nursing student uses their own stethoscope and blood pressure cuff to assess the client's vital signs. The student states they know the client is getting better due to the client's most recent temperature of 99.2°F (37.3°C). The LVN assists the nursing student to perform the daily dressing change. The student notes the wound has a scant amount of serosanguineous drainage and reports that another good sign of progress is that the redness around the wound is still measuring 7 cm × 5 cm × 9 cm.

While in the room, the practical nursing student tells the family they can use the patient's bathroom. The client asks the student if they can bring them extra towels and linens "just in case." The student reminds the client that in isolation, the staff does not bring extra supplies into the room. When the practical nursing student leaves the room, they remove their gloves, then their gown, and leave the room. They then perform hand hygiene for 20 seconds.

1. NGN Item Type: Highlight text

1.4.1 Highlight the findings above that indicate the successful outcomes.

Vital Signs

2

Outcome

The student will demonstrate comprehensive application of critical thinking in managing the care of the client with changes in vital signs.

Scenario

A 58-year-old client is in a hospital's surgical unit 1 day postoperative for colectomy. A practical nursing student is working with an LPN on day shift. Together, the LPN and student check the orders and the student helps to document the vital signs. The LVN documents in the nurses' notes.

Health History	Nurses' Notes	Vital Signs	Laboratory Results	Healthcare Provider Orders

- VS Q 4 hr
- NPO
- BR except OOB TID
- Cough and deep breath Q 2 hr
- Sequential compression devices while in bed
- IV NS at 75/hr in left upper arm

Health History	Nurses' Notes	Vital Signs	Laboratory Results

Vital Signs	0900
Temperature (F/C)	99.5°/37.5°
Heart Rate (bpm)	110
Respirations (bpm)	16
Blood Pressure (mmHg)	146/84 right arm electronic
O_2 Saturation	95% on room air
Height	5'6"
Weight	189 lb
BMI	30.5

Health History	Nurses' Notes	Vital Signs	Laboratory Results

0900: Client has an abdominal dressing to the left upper abdominal quadrant that is clean, dry, and intact. The IV of NS at 75/hr is running without complications in the left upper arm. Client states they are tired today and rate pain currently as 3/10 on a 0 to 10 pain scale.

1. NGN Item Type: Highlighting Text

2.1.1 Highlight the assessment findings that require follow-up by the LVN and nursing student.

Health History	Nurses' Notes	Vital Signs	Laboratory Results

Vital Signs	0900
Temperature (F/C)	100.1/37.8
Heart Rate (bpm)	104
Respirations (bpm)	16
Blood Pressure (mmHg)	146/84 right arm electronic
O₂ Saturation	95% on room air
Height	5'6"
Weight	189 lb
BMI	30.5

Health History	Nurses' Notes	Vital Signs	Laboratory Results

Client has an abdominal dressing to the left upper abdominal quadrant that is clean, dry, and intact. The IV of NS at 75/hr is running without complications in the left upper arm. Client states is tired today and rates pain currently as 3/10 on 0–10 pain scale.

2. NGN Item Type: Drop-Down Cloze

2.1.2 Choose the most likely options for the information missing from the statement, below, by selecting from the list of options provided.

Based on the client's assessment data, the student practical nurse determines the client's potential issues are ___1___ and ___2___.

Indications for 1	Indications for 2
Prehypertension	Bradycardia
Hyperthermia	Tachypnea
Stage 1 hypertension	Hyperventilation
Malnutrition	Tachycardia

Scenario

Two hours later, the practical nursing student checks the vital signs again and documents the findings. The LPN reassesses the client, and then the LPN and the student discuss the potential treatment plan.

Health History	Nurses' Notes	Vital Signs	Laboratory Results

Vital Signs	0900	1100
Temperature (F/C)	100.1°/37.8°	99.4°/37.5°
Heart Rate (bpm)	104	110
Respirations (bpm)	16	18
Blood Pressure (mmHg)	146/84 right arm electronic	148/86 left arm electronic
O₂ Saturation	95% on room air	96%
Height	5'6"	
Weight	189 lb	
BMI	30.5	

Health History	Nurses' Notes	Vital Signs	Laboratory Results

0900: Client has an abdominal dressing to the left upper abdominal quadrant that is clean, dry, and intact. The IV of NS at 75/hr is running without complications in the left upper arm. Client states they are tired today and rate pain currently as 5/10 on a 0 to 10 pain scale.

1100: The client rates their pain at 2/10 and denies the need for pain medications. The client states that their blood pressure is never this high; it is usually around 130/mid-70s, and it is making them really nervous. Their hands are shaking, and they report feeling a little lightheaded.

1. NGN Item Type: Multiple Response Select All That Apply

2.2.1 **Based on the client's current condition, the practical nursing student tells their preceptor the client's priority need will be to avoid which of the following? Select all that apply.**

A. Anxiety
B. Postoperative pain
C. Surgical incision infection
D. Increasing hypertension
E. Deep vein thrombosis prevention
F. Rising pulse rate

Scenario

The LPN and the student remain in the room. The client states, "Really, my blood pressure has never been that high, and my pulse is going up too, I just know there is something wrong. Could something be wrong with the equipment? Could you check everything again?" The LPN tells the client they and the student will check the equipment and return in a few minutes. While obtaining the manual BP cuff, the LPN asks the student about what they can do to ensure that they are obtaining correct vital signs for this client.

1. NGN Item Type: Matrix Multiple Choice

2.3.1 **Use an X for the actions listed below suggested by the practical nursing student that are <u>indicated</u> (appropriate or necessary) or <u>contraindicated</u> (could be harmful) for the client's care at this time. Only one selection can be made for each nursing action.**

Nursing Student Statement	Indicated	Contraindicated
"I need to check the rate, rhythm, and strength of the pulse."		
"Use a manual blood pressure cuff to recheck BP."		
"With a tympanic temperature make sure there isn't a lot of ear wax."		
"Administer pain medications."		
"I should continue to hold the client's wrist while I count the respirations."		
"Count respiratory rate for 10 seconds and multiply by 10."		

Scenario

The LPN returns to the client's room with a manual blood pressure cuff. The LPN and practical nursing student discuss measuring blood pressure and pulse manually. The LVN asks the student nurse what she would include when correctly using a manual blood pressure cuff and taking a pulse accurately.

1. NGN Item Type: Drag-and-Drop Table

2.4.1 Use an X to indicate which nursing student actions listed in the left column would be included in obtaining a manual blood pressure measurement.

Nursing Student Actions	Implementation
Check BP in both arms.	
Use the heart rate on the pulse oximeter for most accurate reading.	
Support the arm at the level of the heart when taking the BP.	
Obtain an extra-large size BP cuff.	
Have the client talk to you throughout obtaining BP to reduce anxiety.	
Count the apical pulse if the radial pulse is difficult to obtain or is irregular.	
Have the client rest for 5 minutes before measuring the BP.	
When taking the BP, deflate the cuff at a rate of 2 mmHg per second.	

2. NGN Item Type: Matrix Multiple Choice

2.4.2 The LPN watches the practical nursing student take a full set of vital signs on the client. Use an X or a check mark next to the assessment findings that indicate successful outcomes.

Practical Nursing Student Actions	Successful Outcomes:
Student uses her thumb to measure the radial pulse	
Student states BP is 128/74	
Client reports their blood pressure and pulse are much more their "normal"	
Student states, "I know what I did wrong the first two times"	
Student turns on the TV loudly to help the client relax	
Student tells the client to "just relax and breathe normally so I can count your respirations"	
Student gently places the probe of the tympanic thermometer in the client's ear and pulls slightly on the pinna back and up	
Student documents "Radial pulse 86, regular, 2+"	

3

Nutrition

Outcome

The learner will demonstrate comprehensive knowledge of care of the client with nutritional needs.

Scenario

The client is a 61-year-old admitted to a surgical floor from the recovery room after colectomy surgery for diverticulitis. The UAP has assisted in settling the client in the room and has placed a pitcher of water on the overbed table.

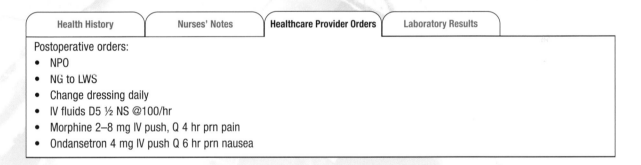

Health History	Nurses' Notes	**Healthcare Provider Orders**	Laboratory Results

Postoperative orders:
- NPO
- NG to LWS
- Change dressing daily
- IV fluids D5 ½ NS @100/hr
- Morphine 2–8 mg IV push, Q 4 hr prn pain
- Ondansetron 4 mg IV push Q 6 hr prn nausea

Health History	**Nurses' Notes**	Healthcare Provider Orders	Laboratory Results

Vital Signs	**1430**
Temperature (F/C)	98.2°/36.7°
Heart Rate (bpm)	96
Respirations (bpm)	18
Blood Pressure (mmHg)	108/50

Nurses' Notes

1430:
- Bowel sounds are absent
- Heart sounds S1S2
- Reports mouth is dry
- Client asks for some of the water
- Client reports nausea
- Abdomen is tender to palpation
- Lungs clear to auscultation
- Spouse says they've been married for 21 years
- Alert and oriented × 4
- NG drainage 50 ml light green fluid
- Dressing to LLQ clean, dry, and intact
- No edema noted
- IV analgesics were administered by the RN in the recovery room at 1345 for pain 9/10 on a 0 to 10 scale, client now reports pain 5/10

1. NGN Item Type: Matrix Multiple Choice

3.1.1 **Place an X to indicate which patient assessment findings require follow-up by the nurse.**

Assessment Finding	Assessment Finding That Requires Follow-Up
Pitcher of water at bedside, spouse asks if client can have some	
Bowel sounds are absent	
Heart sounds S1S2	
Reports mouth is dry	
Client reports nausea	
Spouse says they've been married for 21 years	
NG drainage 50 ml light green fluid	
Pain was 9/10 on 0-10 scale; client now reports pain 5/10	
Pulse 96, BP 108/50	
NPO	

2. NGN Item Type: Matrix Multiple Choice

3.1.2 **Use an X to indicate which two potential issues listed in the left column may place this client at risk while in the hospital.**

Potential Issue	Risk to Patient
Pressure injury	
Dehydration	
Pain	
Constipation	

Scenario

The next morning after report, the practical nursing student checks the orders and documents their assessment.

Health History	Nurses' Notes	**Healthcare Provider Orders**	Laboratory Results

Day 2 0600:
- d/c NG
- Begin clear liquids, ADT

Health History	**Nurses' Notes**	Healthcare Provider Orders	Laboratory Results

Day 2 0800:
Client's bowel sounds are hypoactive in two quadrants and normoactive in two quadrants. Abdominal dressing is CDI. Client's vital signs are stable. Client has been up ambulating in their room and has walked once to the nurses' station down the hall accompanied by a nursing assistant. Client continues to have pain and is receiving IV pain medications from RN with good pain relief. NG has been discontinued. Client reports some slight nausea and states, "I'm not sure I want to drink anything." Client's oral mucosa is dry, lips are chapped, and urine output for the last 2 hours is 80 ml of dark amber urine.

1. NGN Item Type: Drop-Down Rationale

3.2.1 Choose the most likely options for the information missing from the statements below by selecting from the lists of options provided.

Based on the patient's assessment data, the nurse determines the patient is at *highest risk* for _____1_____ as evidenced by the indications of _____2_____

Indications for 1	Indications for 2
Venous thrombus embolus	Walked once to the nurses' station, dry mucous membranes
Dehydration	Dry mucous membranes, 80 ml dark amber urine, chapped lips, slight nausea, "not sure I want to drink anything"
Uncontrolled pain	Continues to have pain, receiving IV pain medication, walked once to nurses' station, slight nausea

2. NGN Item Type: Matrix Multiple Choice

3.2.2 Use an X to indicate which nursing actions listed below are <u>indicated</u> (appropriate or necessary) or <u>contraindicated</u> (could be harmful) for the client's care at this time. Only one selection can be made for each nursing action.

Nursing Action	Indicated	Contraindicated
Bring the client coffee with cream and sugar		
Ask the RN to administer prescribed ondansetron IV push for nausea		
Suggest the client try a popsicle		
Ask the client if she'd like pudding or some plain ice cream		
Encourage the client to start with sips of water		
Bring the client her favorite cream of potato soup		
Ask the client if she would prefer grape, apple, or cranberry juice		
Offer the client clear broth or plain tea		

Scenario

Later that afternoon the client has family at the bedside. The client states since she is starting to feel hungry, the family is going to stay and keep her company while she tries out the new diet. The client and nurse agree to advance the diet to full liquids. The client asks the practical nurse to go over what is allowed on a full liquid diet.

Health History	Nurses' Notes	Healthcare Provider Orders	Laboratory Results

Day 2 0600:
- d/c NG
- Begin clear liquids

Day 2 1530:
- Advance diet to full liquids

Health History	Nurses' Notes	Healthcare Provider Orders	Laboratory Results

Day 2 0800:

Client's bowel sounds are hypoactive in two quadrants and normoactive in two quadrants. Abdominal dressing is CDI. Client's vital signs are stable. Client has been up ambulating in their room and has walked once to the nurses' station down the hall accompanied by a nursing assistant. Client continues to have pain and is receiving IV pain medications from RN with good pain relief. NG has been discontinued. Client reports some slight nausea and states, "I'm not sure I want to drink anything." Client's oral mucosa is dry, lips are chapped, and urine output for the last 2 hours is 80 ml of dark amber urine.

Day 2 1610:

Client states abdominal pain is 3/10 with some abdominal tenderness. Abdominal dressing is clean, dry, and intact. Vital signs remain stable. Client reports has not had a bowel movement but has started passing gas. Denies nausea. Voiding clear yellow urine. Lungs are clear to auscultation bilaterally, bowel sounds normoactive. Family at the bedside, and client states starting to feel hungry, and family is going to stay while client tries out the new diet.

1. NGN Item Type: Multiple Response Select All That Apply

3.3.1 When providing dietary teaching, the practical nursing student reinforces which of the following information? Select all that apply.

    A. "You can have strained vegetable juice if you like that."

    B. "A lot of patients like it that they can have applesauce with full liquids."

    C. "You can be on this diet a little longer because it provides more nutrients than clear liquids."

    D. "Milk products such as yogurt, sherbet, and ice cream are allowed now."

    E. "Foods allowed are now softened by cooking them well and then mashing or finely chopping them."

    F. "Strained soups are going to be OK for you."

    G. "If you like mashed potatoes, they can be ordered for you."

    H. "We can get you some scrambled eggs if they are cut up fine."

    I. "This diet is a step up from clear liquids before we try a soft or regular diet."

Scenario

The following day the client is being discharged. The LVN documents the most recent findings in the client's chart.

Health History	Nurses' Notes	Healthcare Provider Orders	Laboratory Results

Day 3 1100: Discharge orders received. Vital signs T 98.6°F (37°C), P 82, R 18, BP 128/72. Lungs are clear, abdomen is soft, bowel sounds are normoactive, and mucous membranes are pink and moist. Client urinating clear yellow urine; has not had a bowel movement. Client reports pain is 8/10. States is happy to be going home on a soft diet and can have any food if it is mashed up. Client states felt nauseated for a bit after breakfast but isn't worried because it went away. States if feeling that way at home, will go back on the full liquids for several weeks until feeling better. Client states is looking forward to having favorite bread at home, which is the "9-grain with a lot of good nuts and seeds; better than the white bread and butter I had with my scrambled eggs this morning." States spouse already went to the store and got mashed potatoes, very ripe bananas, apples, and a big jar of applesauce.

1. NGN Item Type: Highlight Text

3.4.1 Highlight the findings that indicate the patient is progressing as expected.

Health History	Nurses' Notes	Healthcare Provider Orders	Laboratory Results

Day 3 1100:

Discharge orders received. Vital signs T 98.6°F (37°C), P 82, R 18, BP 128/72. Lungs are clear, abdomen is soft, bowel sounds are normoactive, and mucous membranes are pink and moist. Client urinating clear yellow urine; has not had a bowel movement. Client reports pain is 8/10. States is happy to be going home on a soft diet and can have any food if it is mashed up. Client states felt nauseated for a bit after breakfast but isn't worried because it went away. States if feeling that way at home, will go back on the full liquids for several weeks until feeling better. Client states is looking forward to having favorite bread at home, which is the "9-grain with a lot of good nuts and seeds; better than the white bread and butter I had with my scrambled eggs this morning." States spouse already went to the store and got mashed potatoes, very ripe bananas, apples, and a big jar of applesauce.

4

Medication Administration

Outcome

The student will be able to integrate clinical judgment in assessing, planning, implementing, and evaluating care of the client while administering medications.

Scenario

An LVN is working day shift with a practical nursing student in their first hospital clinical. After checking the chart and assessing the client, they get ready to administer the scheduled daily medications. The LVN asks the student about medication administration as they review the medication orders.

Health History	Nurses' Notes	Vital Signs	Laboratory Results

The client is 32 years old, involved in an MVA late last night coming home from bowling with their coworkers. Client brought to the hospital with a fractured left femur, kept in observation overnight.

Health History	Nurses' Notes	Vital Signs	Laboratory Results

0800: Client cannot remember if they are allergic to anything, states they have no previous health history. Spouse has arrived and is at the bedside this morning, leaving their mom at home to care for their 3-year-old. Client's vital signs are within normal limits. Anticipated discharge home later this afternoon.

---

1. NGN Item Type: Multiple Response Select All That Apply

4.1.1 Which of the following statements by the nursing student require follow-up by the LVN? Select all that apply.

- A. "I know that the peak action of a medication is when it has the highest blood concentration."
- B. "We need to find out if the patient has had any prescriptions before so we can check for allergies."
- C. "The half-life is the time it takes for the medication to leave the body."
- D. "Subcutaneous administration is the fastest absorption."
- E. "I will follow the six rights of medication administration with each medication given."
- F. "My drug book is at the desk so I can look everything up first."

---

2. NGN Item Type: Drop-Down Table

4.1.2 The LVN provides an incomplete list of medications to the student and asks them to complete the information. Choose the *most likely* options for the information missing from the table that follows by selecting from the lists of options provided.

Medication	Dose, Route, Frequency	Indication	Nursing Intervention
Enoxaparin	40 mg SubQ every AM	1	Do not get rid of air bubble in syringe
Influenza vaccine	0.5 ml IM yearly	Prevention of influenza	2
Docusate sodium	3	Constipation	Increase fluid intake
4	5/325 mg one to two every 6 hours prn	Treat pain	Monitor liver function

Options for 1	Options for 2	Options for 3	Options for 4
• Prevents blood clots • Prevents influenza • Treats fever • Relieves pain	• Antidote is protamine sulfate • Not to exceed 3000 mg/24 hrs • Use deltoid muscle • Give in abdominal area	• 2 puffs Q 4 hours prn • 100 mg po Q 4 hours prn • 100 mg po Q AM • 100 units SubQ Q AM	• Heparin sodium • Warfarin sodium • Lactulose • Hydrocodone-acetaminophen

Scenario

The LVN and the student nurse get ready to administer the morning medications. They discuss the medications with the client and the LVN documents the conversation. The LVN and student talk about medication administration and decide to administer the oral medications first, then go back to administer the other medications.

Health History	Nurses' Notes	Vital Signs	Laboratory Results

0830: Discussed with client taking the scheduled Docusate Sodium. Client rates pain on a scale of 0 to 10 at 5/10. Reminded client it has been 5 hours since last dose of pain medication, discussed taking hydrocodone/acetaminophen for the pain. Discussed enoxaparin and offered client a flu vaccine; client accepts.

1. NGN Item Type: Matrix Multiple Choice

4.2.1 Use an X to indicate which nursing student statements listed in the left column may place this client at *risk* while in the hospital.

Nursing Student Statement	Risk to Patient
"I need to check that we give the appropriate drug form and dose."	
"I will double check the medication order to determine if all the required elements are present."	
"If an error is made and is corrected, there is no need to report it."	
"To save time, I'll take the medication out of the original container and place with the other medications in a medication cup."	
"If the client is not quite ready to take the medication, I can leave it for them to take later."	
"I will check each medication with the order three times."	
"Since this is not the first dose of Docusate Sodium, there is not a need to do further teaching."	

2. NGN Item Type: Matrix Multiple Choice

4.2.2 Use an X for the student nurses' following actions that are <u>indicated</u> (appropriate or necessary) or <u>contraindicated</u> (could be harmful) while administering oral medications. Only one selection can be made for each nursing action.

Nursing Action	Indicated	Contraindicated
Asked the client if they want to take all medications at the same time or separately.		
Asked the client if they had any side effects after the previous dose of hydrocodone/acetaminophen.		
Answered another nursing student's medication question while preparing client's medications.		
Used drug book to look up hydrocodone/acetaminophen and Docusate Sodium prior to administration.		
After each medication given, signed off the MAR with the LVN.		
Double checked the correct patient by asking the client if their name is Mr. P.		

Scenario

The LVN and student nurse return to the medication room to prepare the enoxaparin and flu vaccination. After preparing the medications and discussing the administration, they return to the client's room.

1. NGN Item Type: Drop-Down Cloze

4.3.1 Choose the *most likely* options for the information missing from the statement below by selecting from the list of options provided.

When administering the enoxaparin SubQ, the practical nursing student will ____1____, ____1____, and ____1____. While administering the flu vaccination IM, the practical nursing student will ____2____, ____2____, and ____2____.

Options for 1	Options for 2
Give the SubQ at a 45° to 90° angle into pinched up skin	Aspirate for blood prior to injection
Massage site after administration	Perform hand hygiene
Lay syringe and open needle on over-the-bed table while applying bandage	Choose a 23-gauge 1-inch needle to give vaccine
Give injection in abdomen	Inject needle quickly into the muscle at a 90° angle
Wash hands and don gloves	Choose dorsogluteal site for injection

2. NGN Item Type: Multiple Response Select All That Apply

4.3.2 Which of the following findings indicate effectiveness? Select all that apply.

A. Nursing student assesses pain in the client 30 minutes after the oral narcotic.

B. Student applied heat to abdomen after enoxaparin injection.

C. Nursing student identified client using two identifiers prior to giving oral medications.

D. Student states, "It's OK, I don't need to check, I know you now" prior to administering SubQ injection.

E. Enoxaparin given in the abdomen at a 90° angle with a firm quick insertion into the skin.

F. Student states, "I can't see now if the flu shot works, however I didn't see any untoward effects."

G. Nursing student stayed with client while they swallowed their oral medications.

H. Client tells nursing student, "That was a great shot you gave."

Outcome

The student will plan appropriate nursing management and care for the client with mobility needs.

Scenario

A 62-year-old client is admitted to a long-term care (LTC) facility. The LVN checks the chart, completes a morning assessment, and documents an assessment.

Health History	Nurses' Notes	Healthcare Provider Orders	Laboratory Results

A 62-year-old client admitted to a long-term care (LTC) facility for rehabilitation and recovery after a severe automobile accident, fractured left hip and left tibia-fibula fracture. Client underwent surgery and has a long cast on the left leg. Client received a dose of enoxaparin preoperatively and first postop morning. Client was in hospital for 3 days before being transferred. History includes varicose veins in bilateral lower extremities. Client has limited movement and is on bed rest with a trapeze bar. Client is nonweight-bearing, plan for physical therapy to begin working with client tomorrow.

Health History	Nurses' Notes	Healthcare Provider Orders	Laboratory Results

Vital Signs	0900
Temperature (F/C)	99.1°/37.2°
Heart Rate (bpm)	88
Respirations (bpm)	18
Blood Pressure (mmHg)	130/74
Height	5'11"
Weight	224 lb
BMI	31.2

Nurses' Notes

0900: Client's abdomen is soft, nontender, normoactive bowel sound, lungs clear to auscultation, heart sounds S1S2 noted, skin warm, dry, and intact. Client is listless and states that they must get back to work; "what if they don't keep my job?" Client states does not use the incentive spirometer and has refused pain medications and compression device this morning. Client states this facility is about 45 miles from home, spouse will be unable to come often, and client states son is away at college.

1. NGN Item Type: Highlight Text

5.1.1 Highlight the assessment findings that require follow-up by the nurse.

Health History	Nurses' Notes	Healthcare Provider Orders	Laboratory Results

A 62-year-old client admitted to a long-term care (LTC) facility for rehabilitation and recovery after a severe automobile accident, fractured left hip and left tibia-fibula fracture. Client underwent surgery and has a long cast on the left leg. Client received a dose of enoxaparin preoperatively and first postop morning. Client was in hospital for 3 days before being transferred. History includes varicose veins in bilateral lower extremities. Client has limited movement and is on bed rest with a trapeze bar. Client is nonweight-bearing, plan for physical therapy to begin working with client tomorrow.

Health History	Nurses' Notes	Healthcare Provider Orders	Laboratory Results

Vital Signs	**0900**
Temperature (F/C)	99.1°/37.2°
Heart Rate (bpm)	88
Respirations (bpm)	18
Blood Pressure (mmHg)	130/74
Height	5'11"
Weight	224 lb
BMI	31.2

Nurses' Notes

0900: Client's abdomen is soft, nontender, normoactive bowel sound, lungs clear to auscultation, heart sounds S1S2 noted, skin warm, dry, and intact. Client is listless and states that they must get back to work; "what if they don't keep my job?" Client states does not use the incentive spirometer and has refused pain medications and compression device this morning. Client states this facility is about 45 miles from home, spouse will be unable to come often, and client states son is away at college.

2. NGN Item Type: Matrix Multiple Choice

5.1.2 For each client finding below in the far left column, use an X if the finding is consistent with the risk for developing pneumonia, depression, or deep vein thrombosis (DVT). Note each client finding can only be used once.

Client Finding	Pneumonia	Depression	DVT
Varicose veins			
Limited movement & nonweightbearing			
"What if they don't keep my job?"			
Does not use incentive spirometer			
Refused compression device			
Spouse unable to see patient often			
BMI 31.2			
Listless			

Scenario

The next day the client states they do not want any fluids except a little with meals "because it is too horrible to have to use the urinal, last time it spilled everywhere." The client is using the trapeze to change position in bed frequently. The NP discusses the plan of care and asks the client about their varicose veins and BMI. The client reports they are a factory worker and states they stand for long periods of time, and "probably I don't eat well either." After an extensive visit with the client, the NP writes the following orders:

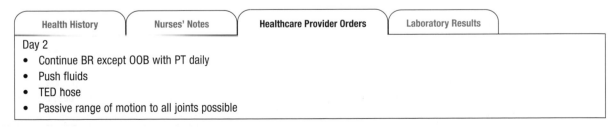

Health History	Nurses' Notes	**Healthcare Provider Orders**	Laboratory Results

Day 2
- Continue BR except OOB with PT daily
- Push fluids
- TED hose
- Passive range of motion to all joints possible

1. NGN Item Type: Drag-and-Drop Rationale

5.2.1 **Choose the *most likely* options for the information missing from the statements below by selecting from the lists of options provided.**

Based on the client's current condition, the client is at the highest risk for developing _____1_____ as evidenced by the indications of _____2_____, _____2_____, and _____2_____.

Options for 1	Options for 2
Pressure injury	History of varicose veins
Fatigue	Limited movement
Deep vein thrombosis	Uses trapeze
Falls	Decreased fluid intake
	Doesn't eat well
	BMI 31.2
	Is a factory worker

2. NGN Item Type: Multiple Response Select All That Apply

5.2.2 **Which actions would the practical nurse expect in the plan of care at this time? Select all that apply.**

A. Encourage the client to deep breathe, cough, and use the incentive spirometer
B. Increase fluid intake
C. Put on the client's TED hose
D. Ambulate three times a day
E. Massage the legs to increase circulation
F. Perform passive range of motion
G. Remind the client that others in the LTC have it much worse than they do
H. Ask the Registered Nurse for a social service referral
I. Leave the client alone as much as possible so that they don't feel bothered

Scenario

The following day the practical nurse arrives on shift to find the client is refusing care. The client tells the nurse, "I don't feel well and can't sleep here." The client states they don't want to do the activity with PT because it hurts too much. The client states they just want to lay in bed. The practical nursing student calls the NP and asks them to visit the client this morning. After seeing the client, the NP writes new orders.

Health History	Nurses' Notes	Healthcare Provider Orders	Laboratory Results

Day 3
- Enoxaparin 40 mg subcutaneous every morning × 8 days
- Hydrocodone/acetaminophen 5/325 one po every 4 hours, medicate prior to PT
- Keep HOB at least 30 degrees for all meals
- Case Management to evaluate
- Please encourage client to choose own meals
- Institute a 3-day sleep record
- Offer incentive spirometry every hour and document
- Nursing to encourage client to perform active (when possible) or passive range of motion to all joints possible each morning and evening

1. NGN Item Type: Matrix Multiple Choice

5.3.1 The NP's orders are reviewed by the practical nurse. Use an X to mark the top three orders that the practical nurse should implement right away in the box on the right.

HCP Orders	Top 3 Orders
Enoxaparin 40 mg subcutaneous every morning × 8 days	
Hydrocodone/acetaminophen 5/325 one po every 4 hours, medicate prior to PT	
Keep HOB at least 30 degrees for all meals	
Case Management to evaluate	
Please encourage client to choose their own meals	
Institute a 3-day sleep record	
Offer incentive spirometry every hour and document	
Nursing to encourage client to perform active (when possible) or passive range of motion to all joints possible each morning and evening	

Scenario

Two days later, the nurse documents the morning assessment.

Health History	Nurses' Notes	Healthcare Provider Orders	Laboratory Results

Day 5
0900: Lungs clear to auscultation, T 101.1°F (38.3°C), normoactive bowel sound, heart sounds S1S2 noted, skin warm, dry, and intact. Cards from family and friends are displayed around the room and the client reports using the tablet spouse provided to send out emails to coworkers and family. Client reports mild left calf tenderness and is performing active range of motion to all nonaffected joints. Client states uses IS every hour and reports "still can't sleep."

1. NGN Item Type: Matrix Multiple Choice

5.4.1 For each client finding, use an X to indicate whether the findings indicate that the client's condition has <u>improved</u>, had <u>no change</u>, or the condition <u>declined</u>. Each row must have only one response selected.

Assessment Finding	Improved	No Change	Declined
Lungs clear to auscultation			
T 101.1°F (38.3°C)			
Cards from family and friends are displayed around the room			
Client reports mild left calf tenderness			
Using the tablet the spouse provided to send out emails to coworkers and family			
Client uses IS every hour			
Client performs active range of motion to all nonaffected joints			
Client reports they "still can't sleep"			

6 Hygiene

Outcome

The student will apply principles of the nursing process and clinical judgment in the care of the client with hygiene needs.

Scenario

A 68-year-old client has been in the hospital for 4 days. After morning rounds and giving morning medications, the LVN returns to the client's room to assess the daily hygiene needs.

Health History	Nurses' Notes	Healthcare Provider Orders	Laboratory Results

A 68-year-old client admitted with acute exacerbation of CHF. History of CHF and hypertension.

Health History	Nurses' Notes	Healthcare Provider Orders	Laboratory Results

1115:

Vital signs stable. Client is on oxygen at 3 L/m, is less short of breath and states still feels a little weak. Client using incentive spirometer. Client is on bedrest except use of the BSC with assist. AM dose of enoxaparin SubQ given. Sequential compression devices (SCDs) are on bilateral lower legs. Client able to move self in bed. Client states, "I just can't do much for myself and I feel really smelly." Last documented bath and full linen change 3 days ago, bed linens rumpled with coffee stain. Client states, "I feel terrible to take so much of your time doing things for me I should be able to do." Client states, "I didn't even have time to grab my toothbrush at home," no toothbrush in the room.

1. NGN Item Type: Matrix Multiple Choice

6.1.1 Use an X to indicate which patient assessment findings require follow-up by the nurse at this time.

Assessment Finding	Assessment Finding That Requires Follow-Up
"I just can't do much for myself and I feel really smelly."	
Last documented bath and full linen change 3 days ago	
Bed linens rumpled with coffee stain	
Sequential compression devices (SCDs) are on bilateral lower legs	
Client moves themselves in bed	
"I feel terrible to take so much of your time doing things for me I should be able to do."	
Using incentive spirometer	
No toothbrush in the room	

2. NGN Item Type: Multiple Response Select All That Apply

6.1.2 Which potential issues may place this client at risk while in the hospital? Select all that apply.
A. Depression
B. Pressure injury
C. GI bleed
D. Deep vein thrombosis
E. Peptic ulcer
F. Immobility
G. Self-care deficit

Scenario

The LVN tells the client they will assist with morning care. The client reports they are very tired and gets increasingly short of breath trying to do anything. After talking with the client, together they decide that a partial bed bath will be the best option for today. The client will wash what they can and the LVN will complete the rest of the bath. The client states they will brush their own teeth and comb their hair, "as long as you don't mind it takes me twice as long." The LVN tells the client that they will get them up to the chair after the bath just long enough to do a full linen change.

1. NGN Item Type: Drop-Down Cloze

6.2.1 Choose the *most likely* options for the information missing from the statements below by selecting from the lists of options provided.

Based on the patient's current condition, the patient's **priority** need will be to prevent _____1_____ while assisting to promote _____2_____, _____2_____, _____2_____, and _____2_____.

Options for 1	Options for 2
Pressure injury	Intact skin integrity
Deep vein thrombosis	A full bath and total linen change every day
Self-care deficit	Client independence and self-esteem
	Hygiene and cleanliness
	Increased client strength by having client do total care alone
	Increased circulation

2. NGN Item Type: Matrix Multiple Choice

6.2.2 Use an X for the nursing actions listed below that are <u>indicated</u> (appropriate or necessary) or <u>contraindicated</u> (could be harmful). Only one selection can be made for each nursing action.

Nursing Action	Indicated	Contraindicated
Warm bath water to approximately 105°F (40.6°C)		
Make sure linens are neat and wrinkle-free before returning client to bed		
Assist the client to put on socks before getting them out of bed		
Ensure the bed rails are up on the side the LVN is not working on		
Return the client to the clean bed and place call light within reach		
Lower the bed height during bath to prevent a fall		
Drape the client for warmth and privacy during the bath		
Allow the client to bathe all areas they can by themselves		
Take off the oxygen while bathing		
Place the dirty linens on the floor on the side that is being worked on		

Scenario

That evening, the LVN gives a shift change report to the oncoming LVN. The new LVN makes assessment and medication rounds. Later in the evening, the client is moving around in bed and cannot seem to get comfortable. The LVN offers PM care.

1. NGN Item Type: Matrix Multiple Choice

6.3.1 Use an X to indicate which actions listed in the left column would be included in the plan of care for this patient.

Nursing Actions	Implementation
Offer a backrub	
Ensure the bed is in the low position with all four full side rails up	
Warm lotion between hands prior to applying to client for backrub	
Ensure the client is comfortable with call light within reach before leaving room	
Remind the client that they already brushed their teeth this morning	
Straighten or replace linens as needed	

Scenario

After providing PM care, the LVN documents the care given.

Health History	Nurses' Notes	Healthcare Provider Orders	Laboratory Results

2215:
Gave backrub with lotion the client's daughter brought to the bedside. Noted deep pinkish-red skin on sacral area. Client states that feels so much better after the back rub; "I think I'll be able to sleep well." Client was provided a washcloth to wash hands and face before sleep. Reminded client the nursing staff will do everything for the client for the morning bath. Bed linens straightened with new pillowcases on pillows. Client's daughter pays a late visit and states, "You smell so good!" Client is resting comfortably with oxygen in place and SCDs on.

1. NGN Item Type: Highlight Text

6.4.1 Highlight the findings that indicate successful outcomes.

Health History	Nurses' Notes	Healthcare Provider Orders	Laboratory Results

2215:
Gave backrub with lotion the client's daughter brought to the bedside. Noted deep pinkish-red skin on sacral area. Client states that feels so much better after the back rub; "I think I'll be able to sleep well." Client was provided a washcloth to wash hands and face before sleep. Reminded client the nursing staff will do everything for the client for the morning bath. Bed linens straightened with new pillowcases on pillows. Client's daughter pays a late visit and states, "You smell so good!" Client is resting comfortably with oxygen in place and SCDs on.

Unfolding Case Study of the Perioperative Process

Scenario

The LVN is working at an ambulatory surgery center that performs outpatient orthopedic surgeries. They are assigned to work with an RN in the postoperative area for the day. The first assignment is K.P. Report from the operating room nurse and anesthesia and is as follows:

| **Health History** | Nurses' Notes | Vital Signs | Laboratory Results |

K.P. is a 62-year-old with a history of osteoarthritis and hypertension. They had a left total knee replacement with Dr. Roberts. They had an endotracheal tube during surgery with general anesthesia. They received cefazolin preoperatively and had a sequential compression device on the nonoperative leg. There were no complications during surgery, incision has Steri-Strips and a silver island dressing applied and then an ace bandage.

| Health History | **Nurses' Notes** | Vital Signs | Laboratory Results |

Patient only responds to tactile stimuli and does not follow commands
Respirations are shallow
Lungs are clear to auscultation
Does not follow commands, so neurological assessment is deferred
Pulses are equal to bilateral lower extremities
Surgical leg is wrapped with an ace bandage and is clean, dry, and intact

| Health History | Nurses' Notes | **Vital Signs** | Laboratory Results |

Heart rate is 110
Blood pressure is 109/67
Respiratory rate is 26
O_2 saturation is 86% on room air
Tympanic temperature is 96.4°F (35.8°C)

| Health History | Nurses' Notes | Vital Signs | **Laboratory Results** |

Test	Results	Reference Range
WBC (m/mm³)	14,850	6,000–17,000
Platelet (m/mm³)	281	120–600
RBC (m/mm³)	680	550–850
Hct (mg/dl)	36	35.0–55.0
Hgb (mg/dl)	13	10.0–18.0

1. NGN Item Type: Enhanced Hot Spot

7.1.1 Highlight or place a checkmark next to the assessment findings that require follow-up by the LVN.
☐ Heart rate is 110
☐ Blood pressure is 109/67
☐ Respiratory rate is 26 and shallow
☐ O$_2$ saturation is 86% on room air
☐ Tympanic temperature is 96.4°F (35.8°C)
☐ Patient only responds to tactile stimuli and does not follow commands
☐ Lungs are clear to auscultation
☐ Does not follow commands, so neurological assessment is deferred
☐ Pulses are equal to bilateral lower extremities
☐ Surgical leg is wrapped with an ace bandage and is clean, dry, and intact

2. NGN Item Type: Drop-Down Cloze

7.1.2 Choose the most likely options for the information missing from the statements below by selecting from the list of options provided.
Based on the patient's assessment, the LVN determines the findings are due to the patient's _____ (1)_____ and sees that it is most likely related to ____(2)____. The LVN also notices that the patient's elevated ____(3)____ is related to this issue.

Options for (1)	Options for (2)	Options for (3)
Heart rate	Preexisting conditions	Level of consciousness
O$_2$ saturation	Too much pain medication	Blood pressure
Level of consciousness	Not enough oxygen	Heart rate

Scenario

After initial interventions were performed on K.P., the LVN reassessed them. The results are documented as follows:

Health History	Nurses' Notes	Vital Signs	Laboratory Results

K.P. is a 62-year-old with a history of osteoarthritis and hypertension. They had a left total knee replacement with Dr. Roberts. They had an endotracheal tube during surgery with general anesthesia. They received cefazolin preoperatively and had a sequential compression device on the nonoperative leg. There were no complications during surgery, incision has Steri-Strips and a silver island dressing applied and then an ace bandage.

Health History	**Nurses' Notes**	Vital Signs	Laboratory Results

Patient is responsive to verbal stimuli, lung sounds are clear to auscultation. Patient denies nausea/vomiting and complains, "My knee hurts really badly." Patient is shivering and appears restless in their bed.

Health History	Nurses' Notes	**Vital Signs**	Laboratory Results

Heart rate is 88
Blood pressure is 128/72
Respiratory rate is 16
O$_2$ saturation is 96% on oxygen
Tympanic temperature is 96.6°F (35.9°C)

Health History	Nurses' Notes	Vital Signs	Laboratory Results

Test	Results	Reference Range
WBC (m/mm^3)	14,850	6,000–17,000
Platelet (m/mm^3)	281	120–600
RBC (m/mm^3)	680	550–850
Hct (mg/dl)	36	35.0–55.0
Hgb (mg/dl)	13	10.0–18.0

1. NGN Item Type: Drop-Down Cloze

7.2.1 Choose the most likely options for the information missing from the statements below by selecting from the list of options provided.

Based on these findings, the LVN determines the priority for this patient is _____(1)_____. The LVN believes the shivering is a high priority because it is most likely caused by ____(2)____. The LVN suggests to the RN that they should make it a priority to implement ____(3)____ to prevent poor outcomes and delayed discharge for the patient.

Options for (1)	Options for (2)	Options for (3)
Administer pain medication	Seizure	Seizure precautions
Pain assessment	Hypothermia	Active warming measures
Notify provider of pain	Malignant hyperthermia	Malignant hypothermia protocol

2. NGN Item Type: Multiple Response Select All That Apply

7.2.2 The LVN collaborates with the RN, and they identify the following care options: (Select all that apply)

a. Administer pain medications as prescribed
b. Administer prn antiemetic to prevent nausea
c. Assess for muscle rigidity, rapid and shallow breathing, elevated body temperature
d. Remove dressing to assess for excessive bleeding and drainage from incision
e. Assess for paresthesia/paralysis, pallor, pulse, pain, and pressure
f. Contact provider to consider loosening the bandage
g. Contact provider to ask for a stat hemoglobin and hematocrit
h. Tell the provider the patient has compartment syndrome
i. Place warm blankets on patient

Scenario

The LVN has been caring for K.P. for approximately 4 hours in the recovery area. They document the following:

Health History	Nurses' Notes	Vital Signs	Laboratory Results

K.P. is a 62-year-old with a history of osteoarthritis and hypertension. They had a left total knee replacement with Dr. Roberts. They had an endotracheal tube during surgery with general anesthesia. They received cefazolin preoperatively and had a sequential compression device on the nonoperative leg. There were no complications during surgery, incision has Steri-Strips and a silver island dressing applied and then an ace bandage.

| Health History | Nurses' Notes | Vital Signs | Laboratory Results |

Patient is sitting up and eating lunch and states the pain is a "2" on a 1 to 10 pain scale. The pain is described as "dull, but it is a tolerable level." The surgical dressing is clean dry and intact. Patient denies any numbness or tingling to extremities. Pulses are 3+ and equal bilaterally. Grip strength and push/pull strength are equal bilaterally. The LVN recognizes that K.P. can get ready for discharge, and the provider writes discharge orders.

| Health History | Nurses' Notes | Vital Signs | Laboratory Results |

Heart rate is 82
Blood pressure is 117/74
Respiratory rate is 14
O_2 saturation is 96% on room air
Tympanic temperature is 98.2°F (36.8°C)

1. NGN Item Type: Drop-Down Cloze

7.3.1 Choose the most likely options for the information missing from the statements below by selecting from the lists of options provided.

The LVN begins preparing K.P. for discharge by _____(1)_____. The LVN also reinforces teaching regarding surgical dressing and ____(2)____. The LVN suggests to the RN that they should initiate ____(3)____.

Options for (1)	Options for (2)	Options for (3)
Remove intravenous access as ordered	Tightens up the ace bandage to prevent swelling and bleeding	Transfer to higher level of care
Gives more intravenous pain medication for drive home	Gets the patient dressed	Discharge teaching
Gives antiemetic for drive home	Replaces the sterile dressing to show K.P. how to do it	Social work consult to prepare for discharge

2. NGN Item Type: Multiple Response Select All That Apply

7.3.2 Choose the most likely options for the information missing from the statements below by selecting from the lists of options provided.

When the LVN is reinforcing discharge teaching, they realize the patient **needs further instructions** when the patient states: (select all that apply)

a. "I need to blow in the incentive spirometer frequently while awake"
b. "I need to eat foods high in fiber because of the opiates"
c. "I can use the hot tub to prevent muscle spasms"
d. "I should take antiemetics every day to prevent nausea"
e. "I should take the antibiotics until they are gone"
f. "I should stay in bed as much as possible"
g. "I should elevate my extremity when I am not walking"
h. "I will go to my follow-up appointment as scheduled"
i. "It is OK to continue smoking"

Chronic Obstructive Pulmonary Disease (COPD)

Outcome

The student will demonstrate comprehensive application of critical thinking in managing the care of the client with chronic obstructive pulmonary disease.

Scenario

The client is a 63-year-old admitted to a medical unit in the hospital with a diagnosis of chronic obstructive pulmonary disease (COPD). The practical nursing student reviews the chart and documents the findings:

Health History	Nurses' Notes	Vital Signs	Laboratory Results

Client has a history of hypertension, asthma, benign prostatic hypertrophy, cholecystectomy 10 years ago, and diverticulitis. Regular medications include tamsulosin, fluticasone inhaler, and lisinopril. Client is divorced, lives alone in a townhouse, and works in a local manufacturing factory. Client currently smokes a pack of cigarettes a day, which client states is down from a high of three packs per day when going through a divorce several years ago.

Health History	Nurses' Notes	Vital Signs	Laboratory Results

Day 1

Vital Signs	0700
Temperature (F/C)	97.8°/36.5°
Heart Rate (bpm)	96
Respirations (bpm)	24
Blood Pressure (mmHg)	132/82
O_2 saturation	91% on RA
BMI	32

Health History	Nurses' Notes	Vital Signs	Laboratory Results

0730 Assessment

Subjective

- Reports has to "get up to pee at night"
- Admits to shortness of breath with exertion and has frequent cough
- States "sleeps on three pillows at night right now"
- States being this short of breath makes them feel jittery and worried
- Reports increased flatulence sometimes

Objective

- Prolonged expiration with pursed lip breathing
- Bilateral wheezes noted throughout
- Scar over RUQ
- 1+ pitting edema bilateral lower extremities
- Pedal pulses 2+ bilaterally
- Abdominal tenderness with palpation LLQ
- Bowel sounds normoactive

1. NGN Item Type: Matrix Multiple Choice

8.1.1 Use an X to indicate which patient assessment findings require follow-up by the nurse at this time.

Assessment Finding	Assessment Finding That Requires Follow-Up
VS: T 97.8°F (36.5°C)	
P 96	
R 24	
BP 132/82	
O_2 saturation 91% on RA	
BMI 32	
Smokes a pack of cigarettes a day	
Client reports has to "get up to pee at night"	
Client reports shortness of breath with exertion and has frequent cough	
Client reports "sleeps on three pillows at night right now"	
Prolonged expiration with pursed lip breathing	
Bilateral wheezes noted throughout	
Client states being this short of breath makes them feel jittery and worried	
Scar over RUQ	
1+ pitting edema bilateral lower extremities	
Pedal pulses 2+ bilaterally	
Abdominal tenderness with palpation LLQ	
Bowel sounds normoactive	
Client reports increased flatulence sometimes	

2. NGN Item Type: Matrix Multiple Choice

8.1.2 Use an X to indicate which top three potential issues listed in the left column may place this client at risk while in the hospital.

Potential Issue	Risk to Patient
Pressure injury	
Constipation	
Depression	
Anxiety	
Congestive heart failure	
Acute respiratory distress syndrome	
Poor gas exchange	
Pneumonia	

Scenario

Several hours later, the practical nursing student receives a report from the Registered Nurse (RN) that the nursing assistant reported to them that the client's oxygen saturation had dropped. The RN put the client on oxygen via nasal cannula at 2 l/m and asks the practical nurse to check back on the client within the next 30 minutes. At that time, the practical nurse documents the following and reports to the RN.

Health History	Nurses' Notes	Vital Signs	Laboratory Results

Vital Signs	1000
Temperature (F/C)	98.2°/36.7°
Heart Rate (bpm)	98
Respirations (bpm)	26
Blood Pressure (mmHg)	132/68
O_2 saturation	90% on O_2 2 l/m

Health History	Nurses' Notes	Vital Signs	Laboratory Results

1000 Assessment

Subjective
- Client reports increasing dyspnea and use of accessory muscles

Objective
- Bowel sounds normoactive
- Slight nausea
- Increasing productive cough
- Fine scattered crackles bilateral bases
- Use of accessory muscles
- 1+ pitting edema bilateral lower extremities
- Pedal pulses 2+ bilaterally

1. NGN Item Type: Drop-Down Cloze

8.2.1 Choose the *most likely* options for the information missing from the statements below by selecting from the lists of options provided.

Based on the client's current condition, the client's **priority** needs will be to prevent _____1_____ as evidenced by _____2_____, _____2_____, _____2_____, and _____2_____.

Options for 1	Options for 2
Acute respiratory distress syndrome	Increasing dyspnea and use of accessory muscles
Congestive heart failure	Slight nausea
Pneumonia	O_2 saturation 90% on O_2 2 l/m
	Crackles and increased cough
	Pedal pulses 2+ bilaterally
	T 98.2°F (36.7°C)
	R 26

2. NGN Item Type: Multiple Response Select All That Apply

8.2.2 The practical nursing student knows which of the following will be included in the plan of care at this time? Select all that apply.

A. Assisting client to prepare for a chest x-ray or CT scan

B. Prepare to administer medications

C. Assisting client to sit up in the chair to support ventilations

D. Monitor for signs of increasing respiratory failure

E. Oxygen therapy to raise oxygen levels as ordered

Scenario

An hour later, the practical nursing student and respiratory therapist continue to monitor the client's respiratory status.

Health History	Nurses' Notes	Vital Signs	Laboratory Results
Vital Signs		**1110**	
Temperature (F/C)		98.2°/36.7°	
Heart Rate (bpm)		94	
Respirations (bpm)		26	
Blood Pressure (mmHg)		134/76	
O$_2$ saturation		91% on O$_2$ 2 l/m	

1. NGN Item Type: Matrix Multiple Choice

8.3.1 Use an X for the three actions that the practical nursing student should perform right away.

Nursing Actions	Actions to Be Performed Right Away
Schedule nursing care to provide for the client's rest	
Teach the client how to perform pursed-lip breathing	
Monitor breath sounds every 1 to 2 hours for worsening lung sounds	
Monitor the client's behavior for signs of restlessness	
Encourage the client to verbalize feelings	
Give handoff to the RN and provide support	

Scenario

Three days later, the client reports to the practical nursing student that they are finally feeling better and "really had a scare." The PCHP has discussed with the client the possibility of discharge the following day.

Health History	Nurses' Notes	Vital Signs	Laboratory Results
Day 1			
Vital Signs		**0700**	
Temperature (F/C)		97.8°/36.5°	
Heart Rate (bpm)		96	
Respirations (bpm)		24	
Blood Pressure (mmHg)		132/82	
O$_2$ saturation		91% on RA	
BMI		32	
Day 4			
Vital Signs		**1300**	
Temperature (F/C)		98.4°/36.8°	
Heart Rate (bpm)		78	
Respirations (bpm)		18	
Blood Pressure (mmHg)		134/78	
O$_2$ saturation		94% on RA	
BMI		32.4	

Health History	Nurses' Notes	Vital Signs	Laboratory Results

Day 4

1300 Assessment

Subjective

- Client reports they can walk up and down the hallway with very little shortness of breath
- Client sleeping with the HOB at 30 degrees without additional pillows
- Client reports still wakes up at least once a night to urinate

Objective

- Productive cough
- No pedal edema

---

1. NGN Item Type: Matrix Multiple Choice

8.4.1 **Prior to discharge, the practical nursing student documents the following information. For each client finding, use an X to indicate whether the interventions led to the client findings improved, no change, or declined.**

Client Finding	Improved	No Change	Declined
Client reports they can walk up and down the hallway with very little shortness of breath			
Productive cough			
Client sleeping with the HOB at 30 degrees without additional pillows			
No pedal edema			
BP 134/78			
HR 78, R 18			
BMI 32.4			
Client reports still wakes up at least once a night to urinate			
O_2 saturation 94% on RA			

9

Cerebrovascular Accident

Outcome

The student will apply principles of the nursing process and clinical judgment in the care of the client with a cerebrovascular accident.

Scenario

A 72-year-old client was moved to a long-term care (LTC) facility after spending 3 weeks in a hospital following a left-sided ischemic cerebrovascular accident (stroke). During hospitalization, they were initially administered recombinant tissue plasminogen activator (TPA) followed by physical and speech therapy. The client continues to have right-sided hemiparesis, weakness, slight facial drooping, and residual speech problems. They are to continue with their rehabilitation with nursing, physical therapy, and occupational therapy. The client's spouse is at the bedside for several hours each day. The practical nursing student assesses the following during their first morning in the LTC facility and documents the findings.

Health History	Nurses' Notes	Vital Signs	Laboratory Results

Day 1

Vital Signs	0930
Temperature (F/C)	98.6°/38°
Heart Rate (bpm)	78
Respirations (bpm)	16
Blood Pressure (mmHg)	138/84

0930 Assessment:

- Alert and awake
- Needs bedrest for several hours after being up in the chair and a short ambulation in hall
- Client states would prefer to stay in bed and not get up
- Left foot push/pull 5/5
- Right foot push/pull 2/5
- Left hand grip 5/5
- Right hand grip 4/5
- Glasgow Coma Scale (GCS) 15
- Coughs when eating lunch
- Spouse states client's speech is "pretty good when it is slow, gets a little slurred if they tried to talk too fast."
- Client reports their legs are "weak and shaky, like they give way when walking."

1. NGN Item Type: Drop-Down Cloze

9.1.1 Choose the *most likely* options for the information missing from the statement below by selecting from the list of options provided.

The assessment findings that require immediate follow-up include _____1_____, _____2_____, _____3_____.

Options for 1	Options for 2	Options for 3
Alert and oriented	Coughs when eating lunch	P 88
"Legs give way"	BP 138/84	Right foot push/pull 2/5
Right hand grip 4/5	GCS 15	"Speech gets a little slurred"

2. NGN Item Type: Matrix Multiple Choice

9.1.2 Use an X to indicate which four potential issues listed in the left column may place this client at the highest risk while in the long-term care facility for rehabilitation.

Potential Issue	Risk to Patient
Fall	
Constipation	
Pressure injury	
Aspiration	
Insomnia	
Pain	
Deep vein thrombosis	

Scenario

Following lunch, the practical nursing student adds to the Nurses' Notes.

Health History	Nurses' Notes	Vital Signs	Laboratory Results

1230: Client was sitting in a chair at the bedside eating lunch and was choking and coughing while drinking coffee. Directed nursing assistant to assist client back to bed. When moving the client from the chair to the bed, the nursing assistant called for assistance as the client's right leg would not support client's weight. Two staff members assisted client back into bed. Client states is exhausted and just wants to stay in bed the rest of the day.

1. NGN Item Type: Drop-Down Cloze

9.2.1 Choose the *most likely* options for the information missing from the statements below by selecting from the lists of options provided.

Based on the patient's current condition, the patient's **priority** need will be to prevent _____1_____ and _____1_____ as evidenced by _____2_____ and _____2_____.

Options for 1	Options for 2
Pressure injury	Client states they are exhausted
Fatigue	Right leg would not support client
Aspiration	Wants to stay in bed the rest of the day
Falls	Choked and coughed with lunch

2. NGN Item Type: Drop-Down Table

9.2.2 After getting back to bed, the client has many questions. For each client question listed below, select the potential nursing response that would be appropriate for the question. Only one option in each response needs to be selected for each question. Note that not all responses will be used.

Client Question	Nurse Response
"Will I ever be able to go home?"	
"When will my leg be strong enough for me to bear my own weight?"	
"Can I just have some coffee without having to thicken it?"	
"If I fall, what should I do?"	

Nurse Response
1. "If you fall and you're not injured, you can roll over and get right up."
2. "A few sips of coffee without thickener will probably be fine, just drink it slowly."
3. "Stay calm. If your caregiver is nearby, have them call for assistance, if not, use your call button or call out for us. Don't try to get up on your own, two of us will help you."
4. "You'll need to follow the plan the speech therapist gives you, right now we are going to thicken all your liquids."
5. "You may need to stay here in the long-term care center for a long time."
6. "It is too early to tell how long it will be before you are strong enough to bear all your weight, but the physical therapists will assist you every day to get stronger."
7. "We'll ask the RN about your plans to go home."

Scenario

At dinner that evening, the practical nursing student reinforces teaching to the client and their spouse for activities of daily living and especially in eating to prevent aspiration.

1. NGN Item Type: Multiple Response Select All That Apply

9.3.1 What nursing actions are appropriate to reinforce to the client and their spouse at this time? Select all that apply.

_____A. Monitor for signs of nausea
_____B. Encourage high fowlers such as a chair for eating and drinking
_____C. Brush the client's teeth and comb their hair to save their strength
_____D. Instruct the client not to get out of the chair after eating without assistance
_____E. Encourage the client to tilt their head and neck back when swallowing

Scenario

Four weeks later, the client and their spouse are excited for the anticipated discharge to their home tomorrow. The Registered Nurse documents care in the client's chart.

Health History	Nurses' Notes	Vital Signs	Laboratory Results

Week 4, 1300: Client will have home health visits from a Registered Nurse for care coordination and from a practical nursing student for help with medications. A nursing assistant will help with personal care, and physical therapy will be continued at home to assist with strength and balance.

1. NGN Item Type: Matrix Multiple Choice

9.4.1 For each client finding, use an X to indicate whether the interventions were effective (helped to meet expected outcomes), <u>ineffective</u> (did not help to meet expected outcomes), or <u>unrelated</u> (not related to the expected outcomes). Each row must have only one response option selected.

Client Finding	Effective	Ineffective	Unrelated
"I am excited to go home with home health and have more physical therapy there."			
Client reports they have had an occasional headache like they often have gotten throughout their adult years.			
Client fell last week while ambulating in the hallway.			
Client has not had any choking or coughing when eating or drinking in the last 2 weeks.			
Spouse states that the client is now able to ambulate independently with the walker and it will be helpful to have at home.			

10

Chronic Kidney Disease

Outcome

The learner will demonstrate comprehensive knowledge of care of the client with chronic kidney disease.

Scenario

A 52-year-old client is admitted to the ED. The practical nursing student checks the chart and documents in the nurses' notes.

Health History	Nurses' Notes	Vital Signs	Laboratory Results

A 52-year-old client with history of hypertension, diabetes mellitus type 2, and end-stage renal disease, current complaints of fatigue, itchy skin, and trouble breathing. Medications include captopril, metformin, insulin, calcium carbonate, ferrous sulfate.

Health History	Nurses' Notes	Vital Signs	Laboratory Results

Vital Signs	1330
Temperature (F/C)	98.4°/36.8°
Heart Rate (bpm)	96
Respirations (bpm)	22
Blood Pressure (mmHg)	160/98
Weight	206 lb

Nurses' Notes

1330 Assessment:

- Client states, "I told the doc that I have fatigue, itchy skin, and trouble breathing."
- Client states, "Wow, usually after dialysis I weigh about 196 lbs."
- Diffuse crackles in bilateral bases
- Client reports hasn't been to dialysis in 10 days
- Bowel sounds normoactive
- Heart sounds S1S2, regular
- Doesn't feel like eating
- Muscle cramps in lower extremities
- Client reports their sister lives in Pasadena
- Skin dry and scaly
- Client states, "I've always liked to play a good game of golf."
- AV fistula left upper arm, positive bruit/thrill
- Hand grips 5/5 bilaterally, foot push/pulls 5/5 bilaterally
- Bilateral 2+ pedal edema
- Client states, "I just don't want to do this anymore, I can't do it, I just didn't go to dialysis."
- Client states, "I'm so tired of this, I don't get why everyone is so upset that I treated myself to a big hamburger twice last week."

Health History	Nurses' Notes	Vital Signs	Laboratory Results	
Lab Test		**Client**		**Normal**
Hemoglobin		**9.2** g/dL		14.0–18.0 g/dL
Serum phosphorus		**7.5** mg/dL		3.0–4.5
Serum calcium		9.2 mg/dL		9.0–10.5 mg/dL
Serum magnesium		2.1 mg/dL		1.3–2.1 mg/dL
Serum cholesterol		**205** mg/dL		<200 mg/dL
Serum potassium		**5.6** mEq/L		3.5–5.0 mEq/L
Serum sodium		136 mEq/L		135–145 mEq/L
Fasting serum glucose		**145** mg/dL		74–106 mg/dL
Serum urea		**103** mg/dL		10–20 mg/dL
Serum creatinine		**5.9** mg/dL		0.6–1.35 mg/dL
Serum uric acid		5.9 mg/dL		4.0–8.5 mg/dL

Stromberg, H. (2021). *deWit's Medical-surgical nursing: Concepts & practice* (4th ed., pp. 1145–1147). St. Louis, MO: Elsevier.

1. NGN Item Type: Highlighting

10.1.1 Highlight the findings in the nurses' notes that require follow-up by the nurse.

Health History	Nurses' Notes	Vital Signs	Laboratory Results
Vital Signs	**1330**		
Temperature (F/C)	98.4°/36.8°		
Heart Rate (bpm)	96		
Respirations (bpm)	22		
Blood Pressure (mmHg)	160/98		
Weight	206 lb		

Nurses' Notes

1330 Assessment:

- Client states, "I told the doc that I have fatigue, itchy skin, and trouble breathing."
- Client states, "Wow, usually after dialysis I weigh about 196 lbs."
- Diffuse crackles in bilateral bases
- Client reports hasn't been to dialysis in 10 days
- Bowel sounds normoactive
- Heart sounds S1S2, regular
- Doesn't feel like eating
- Muscle cramps in lower extremities
- Client reports their sister lives in Pasadena
- Skin dry and scaly
- Client states, "I've always liked to play a good game of golf."
- AV fistula left upper arm, positive bruit/thrill
- Hand grips 5/5 bilaterally, foot push/pulls 5/5 bilaterally
- Bilateral 2+ pedal edema
- Client states, "I just don't want to do this anymore, I can't do it, I just didn't go to dialysis."
- Client states, "I'm so tired of this, I don't get why everyone is so upset that I treated myself to a big hamburger twice last week."

2. NGN Item Type: Drop-Down Cloze

10.1.2 Choose the most likely options for the information missing from the statements below by selecting from the lists of options provided.

Based on the client's assessment data and laboratory results, the practical nursing student determines the findings may be due to _____1_____. The client's lung sounds and increased BP may indicate _____2_____, while the hemoglobin level and fatigue may indicate _____3_____.

Indications for 1	Indications for 2	Indications for 3
Limited mobility	Fluid overload	Anemia
Hemodialysis	Infection	Diabetes mellitus
Noncompliance	Ecchymosis	Headache

Scenario

The client is admitted to the medical unit and settled into the room by the practical nurse. After a discussion with the nephrologist and hospitalist, the client agrees to hemodialysis that afternoon.

1. NGN Item Type: Multiple Response Select All That Apply

10.2.1 Based on the client's current treatment plan, the client's priority needs will be to prevent which of the following? Select all that apply.

A. Hyperkalemia

B. Respiratory acidosis

C. Stroke

D. Acute confusion

E. Fatigue

F. Dysrhythmias

G. Weight loss

H. Insomnia

2. NGN Item Type: Matrix Multiple Choice

10.2.2 Use an X for the nursing actions listed below that are <u>indicated</u> (appropriate or necessary) or <u>contraindicated</u> (could be harmful). Only one selection can be made for each nursing action.

Nursing Action	Indicated	Contraindicated
Provide a high-protein diet		
Assess vital signs		
Tell client they absolutely cannot miss a dialysis appointment		
Remind the client that they won't have to worry about their blood pressure after going back on dialysis		
Monitor labs such as H/H, BUN, creatinine, and potassium		
Prevent fluid overload by maintaining fluid restrictions		
Administer medications as ordered		
Reassess for edema, crackles in lungs, and orthopnea		
Remind client they'll be able to go off dialysis soon		

Scenario

Four days later, the client is stabilized and preparing for discharge after hemodialysis the following morning. They have had 2 days of hemodialysis while in the hospital, and their next hemodialysis at their outpatient center has been scheduled.

Health History	Nurses' Notes	Vital Signs	Laboratory Results

Vital Signs	1115
Temperature (F/C)	98.4°/36.8°
Heart Rate (bpm)	82
Respirations (bpm)	18
Blood Pressure (mmHg)	140/82
Weight	201 lb

Nurses' Notes

1115: Client to be discharged tomorrow morning. Discussed plan with client who reports that they are feeling like they have a little more energy. Client states, "This is still just too hard for me to do every day."

1. NGN Item Type: Multiple Response Select All That Apply

10.3.1 When reinforcing discharge teaching, the practical nurse includes which of the following statements? Select all that apply.

A. "Joining a support group may help you to stick to your treatment plan."

B. "Eat a high-protein and low-potassium diet."

C. "If possible, include your family in discussions about assisting in coping with lifestyle changes."

D. "While on dialysis, you won't need to reduce your sodium in your diet."

E. "Check your weight every morning and write it down."

F. "Plan activities to avoid fatigue."

2. NGN Item Type: Matrix Multiple Choice

10.3.2 Use an X to indicate which assessment findings in the left column indicate successful outcomes for the actions taken.

Finding	Successful Outcomes
Client verbalized understanding of diet and fluid restrictions	
Client's weight is down 5 lbs from admission	
Crackles are noted in posterior lung fields bilaterally	
BP 140/82	
Client states, "This is still just too hard for me to do every day."	
Client reports feeling like they have a little more energy	

11

Diabetes Mellitus Type 2

Outcome

The student will be able to integrate clinical judgment in planning, implementing, and evaluating care of the client with diabetes mellitus type 2.

Scenario

A 56-year-old client is visiting their primary healthcare provider (PCHP) for an annual visit. After performing a physical assessment, the practical nurse documents in the client's medical record.

Health History	Nurses' Notes	**Vital Signs**	Laboratory Results

Vital Signs	**1545**
Temperature (F/C)	97.8°/36.5°C
Heart Rate (bpm)	78
Respirations (bpm)	16
Blood Pressure (mmHg)	136/76
Height	6´
Weight	226 lb/102.5 kg
BMI	30.6

Health History	**Nurses' Notes**	Vital Signs	Laboratory Results

1545: Client states has no previous history and no known allergies. Client states does not take any daily medications at home except a vitamin "when I remember." Client reports increased fatigue and thirst, and also states has to get up to pee at night. Client reports thinks mother had high blood sugars. Works as a clerk and sits "almost all day." States "I will not get a flu shot." Reports bilateral knee pain 1/10 on 0 to 10 scale. Lungs clear to auscultation throughout. Abdomen soft and nontender.

1. NGN Item Type: Matrix Multiple Choice

11.1.1 Use an X to indicate which client findings require further review by the nurse at this time.

Finding	Finding That Requires Further Review
Reports increased fatigue	
BP 136/76	
T 97.8°F (36.5°C)	
Verbalizes has to get up to pee at night	
Lungs clear to auscultation throughout	
Abdomen soft and nontender	
Reports mother had high blood sugars	
States "I will not get a flu shot"	
Ht 6´, Wt 226 lb, BMI 30.6	
Works as a clerk and sits "almost all day"	
Reports bilateral knee pain 1/10 on 0 to 10 scale	
Reports increased thirst	

2. NGN Item Type: Drop-Down Cloze Rationale

11.1.2 Choose the *most likely* options for the information missing from the statements below by selecting from the lists of options provided.

Based on the nurse's findings, the client *most likely* has _____1_____ as the *priority* condition as evidenced by _____2_____, _____2_____, _____2_____, _____2_____, and _____2_____.

Options for 1	Options for 2
Benign prostatic hypertrophy	Fatigue
Osteoarthritis	BP
Diabetes mellitus type 2	Urinates at night
	History of mother's high blood sugars
	Increased thirst
	Doesn't want flu shot
	High BMI
	Bilateral knee pain
	BP 136/76

Scenario

The client was sent to the lab and returned to the PHCP for results 2 weeks later.

Health History	Nurses' Notes	Vital Signs	Laboratory Results

Vital Signs	0920
Temperature (F/C)	97.8°/36.5°
Heart Rate (bpm)	72
Respirations (bpm)	18
Blood Pressure (mmHg)	138/78
Height	6′
Weight	226 lb/102.5 kg
BMI	30.6

Health History	Nurses' Notes	Vital Signs	Laboratory Results

	Client	Reference Range
Glucose (fasting)	142 mg/dL (H)	70–110 mg/dL
Hemoglobin A1c	Client	Reference Range
	7% (H)	< 5.7% normal

Health History	Nurses' Notes	Vital Signs	Laboratory Results	Healthcare Provider Orders
Metformin 500 mg orally twice a day				

1. NGN Item Type: Drop-Down Cloze

11.2.1 Choose the *most likely* options for the information missing from the statements below by selecting from the lists of options provided.

Based on the patient's current treatment plan, the patient's **priority** need will be to prevent _____1_____. Other complications that may develop in the future include _____2_____, _____2_____, _____2_____, and _____2_____.

Options for 1	Options for 2
Pancreas transplant	Crohn's disease
Hyperglycemia	Peripheral vascular disease
Weight gain	Renal failure
	Diarrhea
	Diabetic retinopathy
	Appendicitis
	Diabetic neuropathy
	Increased urination

2. NGN Item Type: Matrix Multiple Choice

11.2.2 The practical nurse is asked to reinforce teaching about home medications. Use an X for the nursing actions listed below that are <u>indicated</u> (appropriate or necessary) or <u>contraindicated</u> (could be harmful) for the client's care at this time. Only one selection can be made for each nursing action.

Nursing Action	Indicated	Contraindicated
"Metformin increases the tissue response to insulin"		
"Make sure to take your metformin every day as prescribed"		
"This medication delays carbohydrate digestion and absorption"		
"You'll need to check your blood sugar as ordered by your PHCP"		
"Insulin may still be needed during times of stress or illness"		
"Metformin may mask symptoms of hypoglycemia"		
"If you need a radiologic study with contrast dye for your knee pain that's fine with taking metformin"		

Scenario

The client returns to the PCHP clinic 8 weeks later for a follow-up visit. The practical nurse reviews the daily blood sugar logs to find the client's blood sugar continues to be elevated most days. The client had labs drawn the previous week.

Health History	Nurses' Notes	Vital Signs	Laboratory Results

Vital Signs	1100
Temperature (F/C)	97.8°/36.5°
Heart Rate (bpm)	82
Respirations (bpm)	16
Blood Pressure (mmHg)	132/78
Height	6′
Weight	224 lb/101.6 kg
BMI	30.6

Health History	Nurses' Notes	Vital Signs	Laboratory Results

Glucose (fasting)	Client	Reference Range
	138 mg/dL (H)	70–110 mg/dL
Hemoglobin A1c	Client	Reference Range
	6.9% (H)	< 5.7% normal

1. NGN Item Type: Extended Multiple Response

11.3.1 When reinforcing diabetes mellitus type 2 teaching, the nurse includes which of the following information? Select all that apply.

   A. "Wash and thoroughly dry and inspect each foot for abnormalities."
   B. "If you are sick, it is OK to skip your medication for that day."
   C. "Remember you need to take your metformin every day as prescribed."
   D. "It is important to check your glucose correctly."
   E. "You do not need to test your urine if you are checking blood glucose levels."
   F. "Long-term complications develop from elevated blood sugars over a long time, so it is important to control your blood sugar levels."
   G. "Reduce your calories and keep the appointment we set up for you with the dietician."
   H. "Increasing your physical exercise can help reduce your blood sugar levels and your weight."
   I. "You may be a candidate for an insulin pump, we can ask your PHCP."

Scenario

The client returns the following month for a follow-up appointment.

Health History	Nurses' Notes	Vital Signs	Laboratory Results

1300: The client brought spouse to visit today. The client's most recent lab draw shows the hemoglobin A1c of 6.4%.

1. NGN Item Type: Matrix Multiple Choice

11.4.1 Before leaving the appointment, the nurse assesses the following client statements. Use an X or a checkmark next to the assessment findings that indicate successful outcomes.

Client Statement	Successful Outcomes
"I'm really proud of myself, I've lost 10 pounds.	
"Taking my metformin every morning has now become a habit."	
"My daughter had her 16th birthday last week and I splurged and had two pieces of cake."	
"I'm having a difficult time exercising so most days I just don't."	
"My spouse encouraged me to join a diabetic support group at church and now we both go."	
"I'm my son's scout troop master, and last week when we had pizza, I just took an extra metformin."	
"My extra glucometer goes with me everywhere in case I need to test my blood sugar."	

12 Inflammatory Bowel Disease

Outcome

The student will use clinical judgment in nursing management of a patient with inflammatory bowel disease.

Scenario

A 52-year-old client is hospitalized after visiting their primary health care provider earlier in the morning. The practical nursing student on the medical unit has been assigned to verify the client's condition and documents the following findings in the chart.

Health History	Nurses' Notes	Healthcare Provider Orders	Laboratory Results

52-year-old client, direct admit from primary health care provider office, chief complaint: not been feeling well for days with increasing abdominal cramping after meals along with diarrhea five or six times a day.

Health History	Nurses' Notes	Healthcare Provider Orders	Laboratory Results

1115
Admit to medical unit
CT scan
IV NS at 100 mL/hr

Health History	Nurses' Notes	Healthcare Provider Orders	Laboratory Results

Vital Signs	1115
Temperature (F/C)	100.2°/37.8°
Heart Rate (bpm)	86
Respirations (bpm)	16
Blood Pressure (mmHg)	108/62
Height	5'6"
Weight	108 lb
BMI	17.4

Nurses' Notes

1130 Assessment:

Subjective:
- Was told several years ago didn't have ulcers in intestines
- Has hot flashes and hot flushes along with some night sweats
- Client states, "Thank goodness I don't have bloody diarrhea, that would be terrible"
- Date of last mammogram 3 years ago
- Client states, "I just can't eat and even drinking water bothers me"
- Lost some weight this past year, states usual weight around 129
- Pain rated 2/10 on 1 to 10 scale
- Client states, "I'm embarrassed by a little dribbling of urine especially when laughing or coughing"

Objective:
- Abdominal distention and RLQ tenderness upon palpation
- Bowel sounds hypoactive
- Skin turgor poor
- Dry mucous membranes
- Urine 100 mL dark amber

Health History	Nurses' Notes	Healthcare Provider Orders	Laboratory Results	

Lab Test	Client		Normal
Hemoglobin	11.2 g/dL		12.0–18.0 g/dL
Hematocrit	36 mL/dL		37–54 mL/dL
Serum potassium	3.6 mEq/L		3.5–5.0 mEq/L

1. NGN Item Type: Multiple Response Select N

12.1.1 Which of the following *seven* findings require follow-up at this time by the practical nursing student?

A. Increasing abdominal cramping and bloating after meals with diarrhea five or six times a day

B. Client states "Thank goodness it isn't bloody diarrhea"

C. T 100.2°F (37.8°C)

D. Weight 108 lb., client reports usual weight around 129 lb.

E. Bowel sounds hypoactive, abdominal distention and RLQ tenderness upon palpation

F. Client states has hot flashes and hot flushes along with some night sweats

G. Skin turgor poor, dry mucus membranes, urine 100 mL dark amber

H. Client states is "embarrassed occasionally by a little dribbling of urine"

I. Abdominal pain rated 2/10 on 1 to 10 scale

J. Client reports "just can't eat" and even drinking water bothers them

K. Date of last mammogram 3 years ago

L. Labs: Hgb: 12 g/dL Hct: 36 mL/dL K+: 3.6 mmol/L

Scenario

Health History	Nurses' Notes	Healthcare Provider Orders	Vital Signs

1345: Healthcare provider notified results of CT scan: thickening in the distal ileus and proximal colon without ulcerations

1. NGN Item Type: Matrix Multiple Response

12.2.1 Use an X to indicate if the findings are most consistent with the disease process of ulcerative colitis or Crohn's disease. Each row may have multiple responses.

Findings	Ulcerative Colitis	Crohn's Disease
No ulcerations seen on CT scan		
Thickening in distal ileus and proximal colon		
Abdominal pain		
Abdominal cramping and bloating after meals		
Bloody diarrhea with mucus		
Weight from 129 to 108		
Thickening and ulcerations in only the colon		
"I just can't eat"		
Low-grade fever		

Scenario

Later that afternoon, the nurse makes rounds and finds the client is tearful.

Health History	**Nurses' Notes**	Healthcare Provider Orders	Laboratory Results

1630: Client states they need to get well quickly and get out of the hospital so they can go to their niece's wedding. Client states they did not think that they would be admitted and that there cannot be that much wrong with them. Client is upset by their NPO status. Client states, "After all, there's not much that can happen to me with a little abdominal pain and diarrhea."

1. NGN Item Type: Drop-Down Cloze

12.3.1 Choose the most likely options for the information missing from the statements below by selecting from the lists of options provided.

Based on the patient's condition, the practical nursing student should first address the client's _____1_____ followed by the client's _____2_____.

Options for 1	Options for 2
Pain of 2/10	Coping skills
Fluid volume deficit	Hot flashes with night sweats
Abdominal cramping	Altered nutrition with weight loss

2. NGN Item Type: Multiple Response Select All That Apply

12.3.2 The practical nursing student anticipates that which of the following will be included in the plan of care? Select all that apply.
   A. Monitor the client for edema and weight gain
   B. Measure intake and output
   C. Monitor stools for number and character
   D. Offer any preferred foods to assist in more rapid weight gain
   E. Assist the client to use self-reported pain rating using the 0 to 10 scale
   F. Administer prescribed oral medications
   G. Recommend client eat a high-fiber breakfast once at home
   H. Assist the RN in administering and monitoring infliximab IV
   I. Reinforce teaching on disease process, complications, and length of stay

Scenario

The following afternoon, the nurse documents in the nurses' notes and reviews the new healthcare provider orders.

Health History	**Nurses' Notes**	Healthcare Provider Orders	Laboratory Results

Day 2
1445: Client states feels "much, much better." Abdominal cramping is subsiding, bowel sounds are normoactive, mucous membranes are moist. T 99.1°F (37.2°C).

Health History	Nurses' Notes	**Healthcare Provider Orders**	Laboratory Results

Day 2
1400: Advance diet as tolerated

1. NGN Item Type: Matrix Multiple Choice

12.4.1 Use an X to indicate which actions listed in the left column the practical nursing student anticipates would be added to the plan of care for this patient.

Nursing Actions	Implementation
Auscultation of bowel sounds every 4 hours	
Offer small frequent bland meals	
Anticipate enteral feedings	
Auscultate lung sounds for crackles	
Report signs of complications such as bowel perforation to RN immediately	
Insert indwelling catheter to measure urine output hourly	
Request a dietary consultation from the RN	
Encourage dairy products to soothe the bowels	

2. NGN Item Type: Matrix Multiple Choice

12.4.2 Use an X for the findings in the left column that indicate successful outcomes.

Findings	Successful Outcomes
Elastic skin turgor, moist mucous membranes	
Abdominal pain rated 1/10 on 0 to 10 scale	
Weight prior to discharge 112	
Client reports was incontinent of urine last night	
T 99.1°F (37.2°C)	
Client reports no abdominal cramping after small bland meal	
Hgb: 10 g/dL Hct: 30.2%	
Urine clear, straw colored	
Stools semiformed to formed twice daily	

13

Heart Failure

Outcome

The student will demonstrate comprehensive application of critical thinking in managing the care of the client with heart failure.

Scenario

The nurse coming on duty to the ED reviews the client's chart from the previous shift.

Health History	Nurses' Notes	Healthcare Provider Orders	Laboratory Results

62-year-old client presents to the ED with increasing shortness of breath, dyspnea, and fatigue. Client states has experienced this a few times over the last year, but this time it "hasn't gone away." Client has history of hypertension and admits "I'm not as good as I should be taking my medications." Client reports an occasional mild cough but denies a productive cough, chest pain, or edema. Client states, "I've been a little more thirsty lately." Client states it has been tough the last couple of days to get meals or even to get to the bathroom. Client reports smoked years ago. Reports sleeping on three pillows for the last week and has been extra thirsty lately. Client's spouse died 6 years ago, daughter lives an hour away, client states they live alone at home. Current medications: hydrochlorothiazide 25 mg po daily, metoprolol XL 25 mg po daily, multiple vitamin po daily, ASA 81 mg po daily, omega-3 supplement po daily.

Health History	Nurses' Notes	Healthcare Provider Orders	Laboratory Results

Vital Signs	1000
Temperature (F/C)	97.4°/36.3°
Heart Rate (bpm)	96
Respirations (bpm)	24
Blood Pressure (mmHg)	162/90
O$_2$ sat	90% on room air
Height	5'3"
Weight	180
BMI	31.9

Nurses' Notes

1000: Admitted to ED bed 3, client alert and oriented × 4, cardiac regular rate and rhythm, lungs diminished in the bases bilaterally with crackles present, abdomen soft and nontender, bowel sounds normoactive, voiding clear, yellow urine, skin warm, dry, and intact, WBC and H/H within normal limits, ECG normal sinus rhythm.

Health History	Nurses' Notes	Healthcare Provider Orders	Vital Signs

1040: Admit to medical unit

1. NGN Item Type: Multiple Response Select N

13.1.1 Use an X for the top *five* findings that would require immediate follow-up.

Patient Findings	Top 5 Findings
BP 162/90; R 24	
History of hypertension	
Lungs diminished in the bases bilaterally with crackles	
Occasional mild nonproductive cough	
Lives alone at home	
Increasing shortness of breath, dyspnea, and fatigue	
Sleeping on three pillows	
O_2 sat 90% on room air	

2. NGN Item Type: Multiple Response Select N

13.1.2 Select the four findings that support the probable diagnosis of left-sided heart failure.

- Client states, "I've been a little thirstier lately."
- Client states, "I'm alone at home now."
- Lung sounds diminished in bases with crackles bilaterally.
- Client reports they smoked a long time ago.
- Visible increased shortness of breath with activity
- Client reports increased fatigue.
- Client states, "I'm not so good at remembering to take my medications."
- Client history of hypertension, current BP 160/90
- Client reports dyspnea.
- Client states, "I'm sleeping propped up on three pillows right now."

Scenario

The following morning, the nurse documents in the nurses' notes.

Health History	Nurses' Notes	Healthcare Provider Orders	Laboratory Results

Day 2
0945: Client's shortness of breath is not improved, O_2 saturations dropped to 88% on room air, started on oxygen at 2 L/m nasal cannula. Client is slightly confused, doesn't remember where she is. Healthcare provider notified this morning's lab results—brain natriuretic peptide (BNP) level 504 pg/mL, and bedside echocardiogram showing left ventricular hypertrophy and an ejection fraction of 43%.

Health History	Nurses' Notes	Healthcare Provider Orders	Laboratory Results

Day 2
0955:
Transfer client to the telemetry monitoring unit
Bumetanide 1 mg po now
Enalapril 5 mg po daily
Continue metoprolol

1. NGN Item Type: Drop-Down Cloze

13.2.1 Choose the *most likely* options for the information missing from the statement below by selecting from the list of options provided.

Based on the client's condition, the practical nursing student determines the priority need is to prevent _____1_____. In addition, they will need interventions to prevent _____2_____ .

Indications for 1	Indications for 2
Immobility	Deep vein thrombosis
Acute pulmonary edema	Social isolation
Pressure ulcer	Right-sided heart failure

2. NGN Item Type: Matrix Multiple Choice

13.2.2 Use an X to indicate which actions listed in the left column would be included in the plan of care for this client.

Nursing Actions	Implementation
Assist the RN with monitoring IV	
Keep the client positioned in fowlers or high fowlers	
Reassess lung sounds every shift	
Instruct the nursing assistant to follow strict I/O	
Administer prescribed medications	
Increase oxygen to maintain oxygen saturation as prescribed	

Scenario

Four days later, the nurse reviews the healthcare provider orders and previous shift nurses' notes. The nurse discusses the findings with the client, who has many questions about going home.

Health History	Nurses' Notes	Healthcare Provider Orders	Laboratory Results

Day 6
0730:
Anticipate discharge home tomorrow if oxygen saturations remain above 92%
Ambulate client in hallway without oxygen and document oxygen saturation

Health History	Nurses' Notes	Healthcare Provider Orders	Laboratory Results

Day 6

Vital Signs	0630
Temperature (F/C)	97.8°/36.5°
Heart Rate (bpm)	88
Respirations (bpm)	20
Blood Pressure (mmHg)	150/82
O_2 sat	94% on 1 L/m oxygen

0630:
Client states is feeling much better and is eagerly anticipating discharge home. Lungs are clear to auscultation; client reports only no or mild shortness of breath when ambulating in the hallway.

1. NGN Item Type: Multiple Response Select All That Apply

13.3.1 When reinforcing teaching, what nursing actions are appropriate for the patient at this time? Select all that apply.

A. Balance your rest and activity throughout the day.

B. Follow the diet as indicated, including lowering your sodium intake.

C. Avoid using the microwave.

D. Treatment for heart failure will be needed for 4 to 6 weeks.

E. Measure your weight every morning, and report any changes to your healthcare provider.

F. Take your medications exactly as prescribed, and make sure to take them every day.

G. Here is a list of worsening symptoms you will need to report.

H. Surgery is necessary and your doctor will be discussing this with you.

Scenario

After reinforcing discharge teaching, the nurse documents the client's response.

Health History	Nurses' Notes	Healthcare Provider Orders	Laboratory Results

Day 6

1030: Following reinforcing of discharge instructions, client verbalizes importance of compliance in taking medications. Client states, "As long as I eat a banana every day, I don't need to worry about missing lab draws for potassium." Client verbalizes understanding that medications and lifestyle changes will cure their heart failure. Client reports feeling stronger but is glad that their daughter will be coming tomorrow to spend a week.

1. NGN Item Type: Matrix Multiple Choice

13.4.1 For each assessment finding, use an X to indicate whether the interventions were <u>effective</u> (helped to meet expected outcomes), <u>ineffective</u> (did not help to meet expected outcomes), or <u>unrelated</u> (not related to the expected outcomes). Each row must only have one response option selected.

Assessment Finding	Effective	Ineffective	Unrelated
O$_2$ saturation on room air 94%			
T 97.8°F (36.5°C)			
Client verbalizes importance of compliance in taking medications			
"As long as I eat a banana every day, I don't need to worry about missing lab draws for potassium."			
Daughter will be coming tomorrow to spend a week			
Client verbalizes understanding that medications and lifestyle changes will cure their heart failure			
Lungs clear to auscultation			
Client reports feeling stronger			
BP 150/82			

14

Systemic Lupus Erythematosus (SLE/Lupus)

Outcome

The student will use clinical judgment in nursing management of a patient with systemic lupus erythematosus (SLE/lupus).

Scenario

The nurse in an outpatient clinic settles a client in an exam room and then reviews the health history and documents in the nurses' notes.

Health History	Nurses' Notes	Healthcare Provider Orders	Laboratory Results

39-year-old client in for a primary healthcare provider (PHCP) visit for recent health changes. Client states had a visit to the OB/GYN for a well-woman check for irregular menses last month; the OB/GYN encouraged the client to go and see her PHCP.

Health History	Nurses' Notes	Healthcare Provider Orders	Laboratory Results

Vital Signs	1420
Temperature (F/C)	100.4°/38°
Heart Rate (bpm)	85
Respirations (bpm)	16
Blood Pressure (mmHg)	122/74

Nurses' Notes

1420:

Client describes a gradual onset of pain and stiffness in the fingers of the right hand, left wrist, and both knees. Client states is extremely tired and yet sometimes can't fall asleep. Client reports some generalized weakness and occasional dizziness. Sometimes heart races a bit and wonders if they've been thinking about their pain and it has been making them anxious. Client states has been "a bit constipated," which is not unusual. Client reports sometimes has an odd red rash that goes away. Lungs are clear to auscultation, heart rate regular, abdomen soft and nontender.

1. NGN Item Type: Matrix Multiple Choice

14.1.1 Use an X to indicate which client assessment findings require follow-up by the nurse at this time.

Assessment Finding	Assessment Finding That Requires Follow-Up
Irregular menses	
T 100.4°F (38°C)	
BP 122/74, pulse 85, respirations 16	
Pain and stiffness in joints	
Extremely tired, generalized weakness	
Lungs are clear to auscultation, heart rate regular	
Trouble falling asleep	
Occasional dizziness	
Red rash	
Abdomen soft and nontender	

2. NGN Item Type: Multiple Response Select All That Apply

14.1.2 Which nursing assessment findings support the patient's probable diagnosis of systemic lupus erythematosus (SLE)? Select all that apply.
A. Pain and stiffness in fingers, wrist, knees
B. Extremely tired
C. Dizziness
D. Low-grade fever
E. Trouble falling asleep
F. Weakness
G. Red rash
H. Abnormal menses

Scenario

The PCHP orders labs drawn, and the client returns to the clinic in 2 weeks. The nurse documents in the nurses' notes and notices that some of the lab results were sent to a national lab and the results are pending.

Health History	Nurses' Notes	Laboratory Results	Healthcare Provider Orders

0915: Client returns to office today for follow-up and report on labs. Client states hands are now puffy, and face is red, dry, scaly, and puffy. Client reports is feeling worse; joints ache and are stiff, and is having trouble getting out of bed most mornings.

Health History	Nurses' Notes	Laboratory Results	Healthcare Provider Orders

Lab test	Client	Normal
Erythrocyte sedimentation rate (ESR)	35 mm/hr	0-29 mm/hr
C-reactive protein (CRP)	11.2 mg/dL	< 1.0 mg/dL
Hemoglobin	11.2 g/dL	12–16 g/dL
Hematocrit	34.6%	37–47%
Anti-nuclear antibody (ANA)	Positive	< 80

1. NGN Item Type: Multiple Response Select N

14.2.1 Based on the client's current condition, the client's *priority* needs will be to prevent which three of the following?
- Chronic pain
- Skin cancer
- Fatigue
- Impaired skin integrity
- Pernicious anemia
- Rheumatoid arthritis

2. NGN Item Type: Matrix Multiple Choice

14.2.2 Use an X to indicate which actions listed in the left column would be included in the plan of care for this patient.

Nursing Actions	Implementation
Reassess body systems	
Ask client about ability to perform ADLs	
Encourage the client to stay at home as much as possible	
Reinforce education regarding lab results	
Provide emotional support	
Remind client not to put anything on face rash	
Encourage periods of rest	

Scenario

The client returns to the clinic in 6 weeks for follow-up. The PHCP received the final laboratory results that had to be sent out to a national lab. The lupus erythematosus preparation lab results came back positive. The nurse reviews the chart for new healthcare provider orders.

Health History	Nurses' Notes	Laboratory Results	Healthcare Provider Orders

Hydroxychloroquine (Plaquenil) 400 mg orally daily
Prednisone 10 mg orally daily for flare-ups as needed

1. NGN Item Type: Matrix Multiple Choice

14.3.1 Use an X to indicate which actions listed in the left column would be included when reinforcing teaching for this client.

Nursing Actions	Implementation
Seek support from family and a support group	
Do not take ibuprofen, always take prednisone	
A balanced diet and exercise are important	
Avoid direct sunlight and use a sunblock with SPF 30 or higher while outdoors	
Avoid acupuncture or acupressure treatments	
Report any illness that feels like the flu if it lasts more than just a few days	
You'll need to come in every few months to check for protein in your urine	

Scenario

Eight weeks later, the client returns for a follow-up visit. The nurse evaluates the plan of care and reviews the chart for the most recent lab results and documents subjective statements in the nurses' notes.

Health History	Nurses' Notes	Laboratory Results	Healthcare Provider Orders

Lab test	Client	Normal
Erythrocyte sedimentation rate (ESR)	28 mm/hr	0–29 mm/hr
C-reactive protein (CRP)	6.1 mg/dL	< 1.0 mg/dL
Hemoglobin	10.8 g/dL	12–16 g/dL
Hematocrit	32.3%	37–47%

Health History	Nurses' Notes	Laboratory Results	Healthcare Provider Orders

0830: Client states, "I've added extra vitamins and iron supplements" and has been a bit constipated. Client states, "I only use mild soap all over." Client reports wears reading glasses more often and states "I wear a floppy sun hat, so I don't have to use sunblock."

1. NGN Item Type: Matrix Multiple Choice

14.4.1 For each assessment finding, use an X to indicate whether the interventions were <u>effective</u> (helped to meet expected outcomes), <u>ineffective</u> (did not help to meet expected outcomes), or <u>unrelated</u> (not related to the expected outcomes). Each row must have only one response option selected.

Finding	Effective	Ineffective	Unrelated
ESR 28 mm/h (0–29 mm/hr)			
CRP 6.1 mg/dL (< 1.0 mg/dL)			
"I only use mild soap all over"			
Client reports has to wear reading glasses more often			
Hemoglobin 10.8 g/dL (12–16 g/dL)			
Hematocrit 32.3% (37–47%)			
"I've added extra vitamins and iron supplements"			
Client states has been a bit constipated			
"I wear a floppy sun hat, so I don't have to use sunblock"			

15

Hypertension

Outcome

The student will use clinical judgment in nursing management of a client with hypertension.

Scenario

A 68-year-old client is in the office for a visit with the primary healthcare provider (PHCP). The practical nursing student assists the client to a patient room and documents the following findings.

Health History	Nurses' Notes	Healthcare Provider Orders	Laboratory Results

A 68-year-old client with a history of osteoarthritis and anxiety is in office for visit with their primary healthcare provider (PHCP) with complaints of increasing headaches. The client's family history includes mother (deceased at age 62) with HTN and stroke and father (deceased at age 79) with prostate cancer. The client has NKMA, and current medications include daily multivitamins and Zyrtec.

Health History	Nurses' Notes	Healthcare Provider Orders	Laboratory Results

Vital Signs	0940
Temperature (F/C)	98.4°/36.8°
Heart Rate (bpm)	96
Respirations (bpm)	18
Blood Pressure (mmHg)	182/105
Height	5'5"
Weight	196 lb
BMI	32.6

Nurses' Notes

0940: Client reports is a current smoker, 1 pack/day, history 65 pack-years (30 years at 2 packs/day, 5 years at 1 pack/day). Client denies current exercise plan and reports left knee pain at rest and bilateral knee pain when walking up or down stairs. Client states runny nose and watery eyes "without the Zyrtec" and has been having headaches almost daily. Reports gets up usually once during the night to urinate. Client speaks quickly, hands either gripped together or fidgety.

1. NGN Item Type: Matrix Multiple Choice

15.1.1 Use an X to indicate which patient assessment findings require follow-up by the nurse at this time.

Assessment Finding	Assessment Finding That Requires Follow-Up
T 98.4°F (36.8°C), P 96, R 18	
BP 182/105	
Height 5'5'', Weight 196 lb., BMI 32.6	
Takes Zyrtec	
Increase in daily headaches	
Current smoker, 1 pack/day, history 65 pack-years	
Denies current exercise plan	
States runny nose and watery eyes "without the Zyrtec"	
Reports left knee pain at rest and bilateral knee pain when walking up or down stairs	
Gets up usually once during the night to urinate	
Patient speaks quickly, hands either gripped together or fidgety	

2. NGN Item Type: Drop-Down Cloze

15.1.2 Choose the *most likely* options for the information missing from the statement below by selecting from the list of options provided.

The nurse recognizes that, based on the assessment data and patient's history, the client is currently at highest risk for complications, including _____1_____, _____2_____, and _____3_____.

Options for 1	Options for 2	Options for 3
Dementia	Stroke (CVA)	Cardiac disease
Kidney disease	Dialysis	Blurry vision
Hypertensive urgency	Nausea	Peripheral arterial disease

Scenario

At the end of today's visit, the practical nursing student rechecks the client's blood pressure at 158/94 mmHg and notes the new healthcare provider orders.

Health History	Nurses' Notes	Healthcare Provider Orders	Laboratory Results

Diagnosis: Hypertension
Metoprolol 25 mg orally once a day
Practice lifestyle changes
Return to clinic in 3 months for follow-up checkup

1. NGN Item Type: Drop-Down Cloze

15.2.1 Choose the *most likely* options for the information missing from the statement below by selecting from the list of options provided.

The practical nursing student recognizes that the client's hypertension is most likely due to _____1_____, _____2_____, _____3_____.

Options for 1	Options for 2	Options for 3
Alcohol use	Diabetes	Sodium consumption
Family history	Obesity (BMI 32.6)	Nocturnal urination
African American race	P 96	65-year pack history

2. NGN Item Type: Matrix Multiple Choice

15.2.2 Use an X to indicate which actions listed in the left column the practical nursing student could anticipate would be included in the plan of care for this patient.

Nursing Actions	Implementation
Reinforce teaching on diet including using sea salt instead of table salt	
Suggest RN referral to nutritional counseling	
Compare BP with prior documentation	
Reinforce teaching on coming to office for blood pressure checks so client doesn't have to monitor at home	
Keep blood pressure log	
Reinforce teaching on how to slowly stop smoking	
Assist in planning to slowly increase daily activity	
Instruct that wine is good for the heart, which can decrease blood pressure	

Scenario

The client comes in for a follow-up visit 3 months later. The nurse takes the client to an exam room and documents in the nurses' notes.

	Health History	Nurses' Notes	Healthcare Provider Orders	Laboratory Results

	Day 1 0940	3 months later 1620
Vital Signs		
Temperature (F/C)	98.4°/36.8°	98.8°/37.1°
Heart Rate (bpm)	96	82
Respirations (bpm)	18	16
Blood Pressure (mmHg)	182/105	132/84
Height	5' 5"	5' 5"
Weight	196 lb	178 lb.
BMI	32.6	29.2

Nurses' Notes

1620: Client reports headaches are gone and has more energy. Client states has more weight to lose but already the pain in left knee is better. The client reports is feeling so much better so is starting to skip daily medication now and then.

1. NGN Item Type: Multiple Response Select All That Apply

15.3.1 When providing teaching about the client's medication, the LPN reinforces which of the following information? Select all that apply.

A. "Staying on your medication is very important, you may be on it for your lifetime."

B. "Maintain your BP log so we can track how well your BP medication is working."

C. "Put this medication under the tongue and leave it until fully dissolved."

D. "If you feel any side effects, let your PCHP know, don't stop the medication."

E. "Don't stop your metoprolol suddenly, it can cause rebound hypertension."

F. "Monitor your blood glucose levels daily."

G. "Make sure you change your position slowly to avoid your blood pressure dropping suddenly when you stand up."

H. "Flushing is a common side effect, so take your medication with breakfast."

I. "Keep appointments with your healthcare provider to monitor your blood pressure."

2. NGN Item Type: Matrix Multiple Choice

15.3.2 Prior to the client leaving the clinic, the LPN evaluates the effectiveness of the plan of care. For each client finding, use an X to indicate whether the interventions were <u>effective</u> (helped to meet expected outcomes), <u>ineffective</u> (did not help to meet expected outcomes), or <u>unrelated</u> (not related to the expected outcomes). Each row must have only one response option selected.

Assessment Finding	Effective	Ineffective	Unrelated
Client states they understand they need to take their medication daily			
Pulse 82			
BP 132/84			
Weight 178 lb., BMI 29.2			
Client states usually has one fast-food or frozen dinner each day			
Headaches are gone and has more energy			
Client states has tried to give up cigarettes, but can't do it			
Client states they will check their blood pressure at home daily			
Client continues to get up once at night to urinate			
Client states will stop taking Zyrtec as it raises blood pressure			

Scenario

The LVN is working on a medical-surgical floor primarily caring for orthopedic patients. Report was received, and the nurse decides to see AB first.

Health History	Nurses' Notes	Vital Signs	Medication Record

AB is a 67-year-old who underwent a right total hip arthroplasty 3 days ago. Patient has a history of smoking, emphysema, and non-insulin-dependent type 2 diabetes. Also has a history of osteoporosis, which is not being treated.

Health History	Nurses' Notes	Vital Signs	Medication Record

Upon entering the room, the patient is resting quietly in their bed in no apparent distress. The patient's sequential compression devices (SCDs) are lying on the floor at the foot of the bed. The patient states they have not been out of bed since surgery except to use the restroom.

Health History	Nurses' Notes	Vital Signs	Medication Record

Temperature (F/C)	97.6°/36.4°
Respirations (bpm)	26
Blood pressure (bpm)	176/98
SPO$_2$	**89% on room air**
Finger stick blood sugar	101 mg/dL (normal range 70–110)

Health History	Nurses' Notes	Vital Signs	Medication Orders

Advair Diskus 500/50 1 inhalation twice each day
Premarin 1.25 mg by mouth once each day
Multivitamin with ferrous sulfate two by mouth each day
Docusate sodium 100 mg by mouth twice each day
Oxycodone/acetaminophen 5/325 1 by mouth every 6 hours as needed for pain

1. NGN Item Type: Drop-Down Cloze

16.1.1 Choose the *most likely options* for the information missing from the statement below by selecting from the list of options provided.

The assessment findings that require **immediate** follow-up include _____1_____, _____2_____, and _____3_____.

Options for 1	Options for 2	Options for 3
Type 2 diabetes	BP 176/98	Osteoporosis
SPO$_2$ 89%	Advair	Has not been out of bed except to use the bathroom
SCDs are lying on the floor	Prn pain medications	Docusate sodium

2. NGN Item Type: Multiple Response Select All That Apply

16.1.2 The LVN recognizes AB is at risk for deep vein thrombosis based on which of the following findings? Select all that apply.

    A. 67 year-old on Premarin

    B. Right total hip arthroplasty 3 days ago

    C. History of smoking and emphysema

    D. Non-insulin-dependent type 2 diabetes

    E. History of osteoporosis that is not getting treated

    F. Temperature 97.6°F (36.4°C), respirations 26, blood pressure 176/98, SPO_2 89%

    G. Has not been out of bed since surgery, except to use the bathroom

    H. Advair for emphysema

    I. Multivitamin with ferrous sulfate

    J. Sequential compression devices are lying on the floor at the foot of the bed

Scenario

The LVN discusses AB's potential deep vein thrombosis with the registered nurse, and the physician is notified immediately. The physician wants to do some tests on the patient and put orders in the computer to confirm or rule out the presence of a deep vein thrombosis.

Health History	Nurses' Notes	Vital Signs	Medication Record

AB is a 67-year-old who underwent a right total hip arthroplasty 3 days ago. The patient has a history of smoking, emphysema, and non-insulin-dependent type 2 diabetes. Also has a history of osteoporosis, which is not being treated.

Health History	**Nurses' Notes**	Vital Signs	Medication Record

Pedal pulses 3+ and equal bilaterally, capillary refill is less than 2 seconds bilaterally, hip dressing has scant drainage. The right leg is warm and red with a calf circumference larger on the right than left. The patient has been doing ankle range of motion frequently, but admits to noncompliance with SCDs and physical therapy exercises.

Health History	Nurses' Notes	**Vital Signs**	Medication Record

Temperature (F/C)	97.6°/36.4°
Respirations (bpm)	26
Blood pressure (bpm)	176/98
SPO_2	**89% on room air**
Finger stick blood sugar	101 mg/dL (normal range 70–110)

Health History	Nurses' Notes	Vital Signs	**Medication Orders**

Advair Diskus 500/50 mcg 1 inhalation twice each day
Premarin 1.25 mg by mouth once each day
Multivitamin with ferrous sulfate two by mouth each day
Docusate sodium 100 mg by mouth twice each day
Oxycodone/acetaminophen 5/325 mg 1 by mouth every 6 hours as needed for pain

1. NGN Item Type: Drop-Down Cloze

16.2.1 Choose the *most likely options* for the information missing from the statements below by selecting from the list of options provided.

The LVN is concerned with the patient's potential deep vein thrombus because it may mobilize and become a ____1____. In order to monitor this risk, the LVN understands the patient's ____2____ are early signs of this. If the LVN notices signs of ____3____, they will make sure the RN and provider are notified immediately.

Options for 1	Options for 2	Options for 3
Hemorrhagic stroke	ECG, heart tones	Shortness of breath
Fat embolism	Respirations, lung sounds, SPO$_2$	Elevated PT/PTT and INR
Pulmonary embolism	PT/PTT and INR	Hip pain

2. NGN Item Type: Drop-Down Cloze

16.2.2 Choose the most likely options for the information missing from the statements below by selecting from the list of options provided.

When planning care for the patient, the LVN looks through the physician orders and prioritizes the order for a ____1____ for the suspected deep vein thrombosis. They will make sure there is also an order for a ____2____ to help the physician diagnose the complication. If these tests are positive, then the LVN and RN anticipate the physician will start the patient on an ____3____.

Options for 1	Options for 2	Options for 3
Chest x-ray	Hemoglobin/hematocrit	Analgesic
CT scan	PT/PTT	Anti-inflammatory
Leg vein ultrasound	Quantitative D-dimer	Anticoagulant

Scenario

AB was diagnosed with DVT in the right leg by ultrasound and was immediately started on anticoagulant therapy. After 7 days of treatment in the hospital and further monitoring and testing, the doctor feels like the clot is stable and the patient can be discharged on oral medications.

Health History	Nurses' Notes	Vital Signs	Medication Record

AB is a 67-year-old who underwent a right total hip arthroplasty 3 days ago. The patient has a history of smoking, emphysema, and non-insulin-dependent type 2 diabetes. Also has a history of osteoporosis, which is not being treated.

Health History	Nurses' Notes	Vital Signs	Medication Record

Pedal pulses 3+ and equal bilaterally, capillary refill is less than 2 seconds bilaterally, hip dressing is clean, dry, and intact. The right leg is warm and red with a calf circumference larger on the right than left. The patient has been doing ankle range of motion frequently, wears SCDs while in bed or up in a chair. Patient is ambulating in the hall with physical therapy twice each day and is up to bathroom independently.

Health History	Nurses' Notes	Vital Signs	Medication Record

Temperature (F/C)	98.9°/37.2°
Respirations (bpm)	14
Heart Rate (bpm)	80
Blood pressure (bpm)	118/72
SPO$_2$	**97% on room air**
Finger stick blood sugar	981 mg/dL (normal range 70–110)

Health History	Nurses' Notes	Vital Signs	Medication Orders

Advair Diskus 500/50 mcg 1 inhalation twice each day
Premarin 1.25 mg by mouth once each day
Multivitamin with ferrous sulfate two by mouth each day
Docusate sodium 100 mg by mouth twice each day
Coumadin (warfarin) 5 mg by mouth each morning at 9 am
Oxycodone/acetaminophen 5/325 mg 1 by mouth every 6 hours as needed for pain

1. NGN Item Type: Matrix Multiple Choice

16.3.1 Use an X for the health teaching below that is <u>indicated</u> (appropriate or necessary) or <u>contraindicated</u> (could be harmful) before the client's discharge at this time.

The LVN reinforces health teaching in preparation for her discharge.

Health Teaching	Indicated	Contraindicated
Encourage ambulation as tolerated		
Apply warm packs to right leg		
Massage calf muscle on right leg		
Encourage increase in fluid intake		
Apply compressing stockings as ordered		
Sit with legs crossed		
Eat plenty of spinach, kale, broccoli		
Encourage sitting most of the day		
Take anticoagulants as prescribed		

2. NGN Item Type: Multiple Response Select All That Apply

16.3.2 When the LVN reinforces discharge teaching, they realize the patient <u>understands</u> their instructions when the patient states: Select all that apply

A. "I should take my anticoagulants as prescribed."
B. "It is OK to take over-the-counter aspirin instead of other pain pills."
C. "If I feel short of breath, I should lie down and rest."
D. "I should follow up with my physician to monitor the blood thinner."
E. "I should call 9-1-1 if I get chest pain or tightness in my chest."
F. "I will be on anticoagulants for 3 to 12 months."

17 Parkinson's Disease

Outcome

The student will use clinical judgment in nursing management of a patient with Parkinson's disease.

Scenario

A 69-year-old client has been admitted to a long-term care (LTC) facility. The practical nursing student settles the client in the room and documents in the chart.

Health History	Nurses' Notes	Healthcare Provider Orders	Vital Signs

69-year-old client admitted with advancing Parkinson's disease. Client is married and retired early from job at a local bank. Client has a history of benign prostatic hypertrophy, old back injury, and hypertension. The client regularly takes tamsulosin and metoprolol but has not been taking any medications for Parkinson's disease.

Health History	Nurses' Notes	Healthcare Provider Orders	Vital Signs

Vital Signs	1030
Temperature (F/C)	99.1°/37.2°
Heart Rate (bpm)	84
Respirations (bpm)	16
Blood Pressure (mmHg)	128/72

Nurses' Notes

1030: Client states doctor thinks he has had Parkinson's for a while but that it must have been mild enough until recently that he did not realize that he had anything seriously wrong. Client is slow to get up out of a chair or bed, and reports "back doesn't bother me too much most of the time." Noted jerky start and stop of the elbows bilaterally when trying to bend. Index fingers and thumbs roll together on both hands. Client wears bilateral hearing aids. Heart sounds S1S2 noted, lungs clear to auscultation, abdomen soft and nontender. Shuffling steps and stooped position noted. Client states has some hesitancy when voiding and bladder never feels quite empty. Client states his blood pressure is up, "especially after I try to walk very far."

1. NGN Item Type: Matrix Multiple Choice

17.1.1 Use an X to indicate which patient assessment findings require follow-up by the nurse at this time.

Assessment Finding	Assessment Finding That Requires Follow-Up
VS: T 99.1°F (37.2°C), P 84 , R 16 , BP 128/72	
Client is slow to get up out of a chair or bed	
Client reports "back doesn't bother me too much most of the time"	
Jerky start and stop of the elbows bilaterally when trying to bend	
Index fingers and thumbs roll together on both hands	
Shuffling steps and stooped position	
Client wears bilateral hearing aids	
Hesitancy when voiding	
Client states his blood pressure is up, "especially after I try to walk very far"	
Client states bladder never feels quite empty	

2. NGN Item Type: Drop-Down Cloze

17.1.2 Choose the *most likely* options for the information missing from the statement below by selecting from the list of options provided.

Based on the assessment data and patient's history, the practical nursing student determines the client's slow movement is most likely due to _____1_____, while the client's pill rolling is most likely a kind of _____2_____. The client's cog-wheel jerky movements are from his _____3_____.

Options for 1	Options for 2	Options for 3
Age 69	Muscle spasm	Medications
Bradykinesia	Seizure	Rigidity
Back pain	Tremor	Stroke

Scenario

Client states they recently "began to have trouble swallowing pills and coughs sometimes when they drink water." The client states that their legs have grown weaker, and they have started having difficulty caring for themself such as brushing their teeth and doing up the buttons on their shirt. They are discouraged that they need to come to the long-term care facility but state they know "it doesn't have to be forever, just until I get a little stronger and learn how to deal with all of this better."

1. NGN Item Type: Multiple Response Select All That Apply

17.2.1 The practical nursing student anticipates that when care is planned for this client, for which priority complication will the nurse monitor? Select all that apply.
  A. Falls
  B. Deep vein thrombosis
  C. Pneumonia
  D. Fecal impaction
  E. Aspiration
  F. Self-care deficit
  G. Heartburn
  H. Stress ulcer

2. NGN Item Type: Matrix Multiple Choice

17.2.2 Use an X for the nursing actions listed below that are <u>indicated</u> (appropriate or necessary) or <u>contraindicated</u> (could be harmful) for the client's care at this time. Only one selection can be made for each nursing action.

Nursing Action	Indicated	Contraindicated
Teach client to imagine stepping over something		
Check safety of the client's room for loose rugs and ensure grab bars are placed		
Choose the client's clothing to assist in faster dressing		
Remind client to tuck chin when swallowing		
Instruct nursing assistant to do a total feed to minimize spilling		
Focus on client's abilities and assist as needed with bathing, grooming, and dressing		
Assist client with use of cane or walker as needed		

Scenario

Two days later, the client has settled into their room and the routine of the LTC facility. The client is eager to do all that they can so that they can be discharged home as soon as possible. The client states they missed caring for their plants on the patio and seeing their dog. The client begins to ask more questions about their progress and asks the practical nursing student about their medications.

1. NGN Item Type: Matrix Multiple Choice

17.3.1 Use an X to indicate which teaching listed in the left column would be reinforced by the practical nursing student for this client.

Nursing Actions	Implementation
Carbidopa-levodopa may turn your urine dark.	
Take your Parkinson's medications at the same time each day.	
Take your anticholinergic medications on an empty stomach.	
Some medications you'll be taking for your Parkinson's may initially cause drowsiness, so move cautiously.	
Diarrhea may be a concern with anticholinergic medications.	
The dose of Sinemet (levodopa and carbidopa) will be increased slowly until symptom control is achieved.	

Scenario

Three weeks later, the client is due to be discharged home. The client and their spouse are excited about leaving the LTC facility.

1. NGN Item Type: Multiple Response Select All That Apply

17.4.1 The practical nursing student monitors the effectiveness of actions. Which of the following findings indicate effectiveness for this client? Select all that apply.
   A. Client frequently does not use a walker when ambulating.
   B. Spouse reports that the client can dress themselves with minimal assistance.
   C. Client feeds themselves safely and effectively without aspiration.
   D. Client states, "I asked the nursing assistant to do a complete bed bath for me this morning because it is just so much faster for them to do it."
   E. The client has remained free from falls.
   F. Client states, "I sit upright when I eat and use a straw when I drink."
   G. Nurse notes the client watches their feet carefully when walking.
   H. Client states, "I'm drinking extra fluids now to help prevent constipation."

18

Peptic Ulcer

Outcome

The student will apply principles of the nursing process and clinical judgment in the care of the client with peptic ulcer disease.

Scenario

A 54-year-old client has come into their family practice clinic for a yearly checkup with their primary healthcare provider (PHCP). The practical nurse settles the client in an exam room and documents in the client's chart.

Health History	Nurses' Notes	Healthcare Provider Orders	Vital Signs

A 54-year-old client comes to the PCHP office with a complaint of not feeling well, mostly with pain in the abdomen. Client works as a lawyer and is recently divorced. History includes recent diagnosis of hypertension, for which the client was started on medication and encouraged with lifestyle changes such as exercise and a low-sodium diet. Client states "gave up smoking a long time ago." Medications include lisinopril 20 mg daily, daily vitamin, and ibuprofen several times a day.

Health History	Nurses' Notes	Healthcare Provider Orders	Laboratory Results

Vital Signs	1300
Temperature (F/C)	98.4°/36.8°
Heart Rate (bpm)	86
Respirations (bpm)	14
Blood Pressure (mmHg)	132/78
Height	6'0"
Weight	202 lb.

Nurses' Notes

1300 Assessment:

Subjective:

Client reports
- "I have this pain, it's burning, in the middle of my upper abdomen"
- "Pain in my gut often wakes me up at night"
- "I've tried to eat healthier foods, but I most often eat on the run these days"
- "Work is very busy, I'm often at the office 10 to 12 hours a day"
- "My dad has BPH"
- "This pain in my abdomen is relieved by food usually, so I snack a lot"
- "I'm going to the gym maybe once a week but often I don't go at all"

Objective:
- Stiffness in knees with active range of motion
- New nicotine stains on right hand
- Lungs clear, heart sounds
- Abdomen soft and nondistended
- Bowel sounds normoactive

1. NGN Item Type: Highlight Text

18.1.1 Highlight the assessment findings that require follow-up by the nurse.

Health History	Nurses' Notes	Healthcare Provider Orders	Vital Signs

A 54-year-old client comes to the PCHP office with a complaint of not feeling well, mostly with pain in the abdomen. Client works as a lawyer and is recently divorced. History includes recent diagnosis of hypertension, for which client was started on medication and encouraged with lifestyle changes such as exercise and a low-sodium diet. Client states "gave up smoking a long time ago." Medications include lisinopril 20 mg daily, daily vitamin, and ibuprofen several times a day.

Health History	Nurses' Notes	Healthcare Provider Orders	Laboratory Results

Vital Signs	1300
Temperature (F/C)	98.4°/36.8°
Heart Rate (bpm)	86
Respirations (bpm)	14
Blood Pressure (mmHg)	132/78
Height	6'0"
Weight	202 lb.

Nurses' Notes

1300 Assessment:

Subjective:

 Client reports
- "I have this pain, it's burning, in the middle of my upper abdomen"
- "Pain in my gut often wakes me up at night"
- "I've tried to eat healthier foods, but I most often eat on the run these days"
- "Work is very busy, I'm often at the office 10 to 12 hours a day"
- "My dad has BPH"
- "This pain in my abdomen is relieved by food usually, so I snack a lot"
- "I'm going to the gym maybe once a week but often I don't go at all"

Objective:
- Stiffness in knees with active range of motion
- New nicotine stains on right hand
- Lungs clear, heart sounds
- Abdomen soft and nondistended
- Bowel sounds normoactive

2. NGN Item Type: Multiple Response Select All That Apply

18.1.2 Which nursing assessment findings support the client's probable diagnosis of peptic ulcer? Select all that apply.

A. Abdominal pain, often wakes up at night
B. Abdomen soft and nondistended
C. Works 10 to 12 hours a day
D. Abdominal pain is relieved by food
E. BP 132/78
F. New nicotine stains on right hand
G. Ibuprofen several times a day
H. Dad has BPH

Scenario

One week later, the client returns to their PHCP after having had labs drawn and an endoscopy for the abdominal pain. The PHCP diagnoses the client with a peptic ulcer.

Health History	Nurses' Notes	Healthcare Provider Orders	**Laboratory Results**

Lab test	Client	Normal
Hemoglobin	14 g/dL	14.0–18.0 g/dL
Hematocrit	42 mL/dL	37.0-54.0 mL/dL
Gastric biopsy *H. pylori*	Positive	Negative

Health History	Nurses' Notes	**Healthcare Provider Orders**	Laboratory Results

Esomeprazole 40 mg orally daily × 14 days
Amoxicillin 1000 mg orally twice daily × 10 days
Clarithromycin 500 mg orally twice daily × 10 days

1. NGN Item Type: Drop-Down Rationale

18.2.1 Choose the *most likely options* for the information missing from the statements below by selecting from the lists of options provided.

Based on the client's presentation, the practical nurse determines the priority need will be to prevent _____1_____, which is indicated by _____2_____ and _____3_____.

Indications for 1	Indications for 2	Indications for 3
Physiological stress ulcer	Hematemesis	Elevated BP
GI bleeding	Fatty stool	Pain before meals
Gastritis	Constipation	Maroon bloody stools

2. NGN Item Type: Matrix Multiple Choice

18.2.2 Use an X to indicate which actions listed in the left column the practical nurse will anticipate being included in the plan of care for this patient.

Nursing Actions	Implementation
Reinforce teaching such as avoiding alcohol, increasing rest, and avoiding NSAIDs	
Ask PHCP for referral for nutritional counseling	
Obtain stool specimen for fecal *H. pylori*	
Encourage stress reduction	
Suggest client eat three meals a day to decrease gastric acid	
Discuss smoking with client, and suggest methods to quit	
Reinforce teaching on triple-therapy medications	

Scenario

Two weeks later, the client returns to their PHCP for a follow-up visit. The PHCP reminds the client that their endoscopy did show *H. pylori*, but it did not show signs of ulcerations or bleedings.

Health History	Nurses' Notes	Healthcare Provider Orders	Laboratory Results

Vital Signs	0800
Temperature (F/C)	98.4°/36.8°
Heart Rate (bpm)	72
Respirations (bpm)	16
Blood Pressure (mmHg)	130/80
Weight	198

Nurses' Notes

0800: Client states is starting to feel better with less pain in the abdomen and is not waking up at night. Client is using nicotine gum and enjoying a high-caffeine energy drink before going into court in the morning. Client states is going to Washington state for work next week. Client reports is trying to cut back on long work days and occasionally goes for a short walk at lunch but states it is hard because of the increase in sneezing from the grass growing this time of year. Client admits sometimes forgetting to take their medications.

1. NGN Item Type: Multiple Response Select All That Apply

18.3.1 **What nursing actions are appropriate for the patient at this time? Select all that apply.**
   A. Assist client in finding methods to decrease stress such as mindful meditation.
   B. Reinforce continued need for frequent small bland meals while healing.
   C. Remind client they will need to be seen frequently for monitoring their CBC.
   D. Ask the client to measure their weight daily.
   E. Provide written materials on managing peptic ulcer disease at home.
   F. Remind client that it is now OK for them to consume alcoholic and caffeinated beverages.
   G. Reassess lung and bowel sounds.
   H. Encourage client to continue using Nicorette gum for smoking cessation.
   I. Encourage verbalization of concerns and questions.

2. NGN Item Type: Matrix Multiple Choice

18.3.2 **For each assessment finding, use an X to indicate whether the interventions were effective (helped to meet expected outcomes), ineffective (did not help to meet expected outcomes), or unrelated (not related to the expected outcomes). Only one selection can be made for each row.**

Assessment Finding	Effective	Ineffective	Unrelated
BP 130/80			
Using nicotine gum			
"Starting to feel better with less pain"			
Weight 198			
Sometimes is forgetting to take medications			
Client is going to Washington state			
Drinking more caffeine			
Sneezing from grasses outside			
Cutting back on long work days			
Reports not waking up at night			

19

Pneumonia

Learning Outcome

The student will be able to integrate clinical judgment in planning, implementing, and evaluating care of the client with pneumonia.

Scenario

A 25-year-old client with a history of asthma since childhood is admitted to the emergency department. Client states they have been working pretty hard lately with very little time to even stop to drink enough fluids. The client reports there was a large work gathering 8 days ago. The practical nursing student notes that the client pauses between words while speaking. The nurse documents the following findings:

Health History	Nurses' Notes	Diagnostics	Laboratory Results	Healthcare Provider Orders

1130:
- Reports chills and pleuritic pain
- Auscultation—crackles at bases bilaterally
- Mild shortness of breath noted with activity
- Cough with increased sputum production
- VS: T 101.8°F (38.8°C), P 92, R 22, BP 118/70
- Increased fatigue
- Reports feels achy
- States mild nausea
- Reports tearing in left eye with "gunky stuff"
- Reports eye itchy and uncomfortable
- Takes vitamins and "very rarely needs to use an inhaler"

1. NGN Item Type: Matrix Multiple Choice

19.1.1 Use an X to indicate which patient assessment findings require follow-up by the nurse at this time.

Patient Findings	Assessment Finding That Requires Follow-Up
Reports chills, pleuritic pain, and cough with increased sputum production	
Auscultation—crackles at bases bilaterally	
A little shortness of breath noted with activity	
T 101.8°F (38.8°C)	
P 92	
R 22	
BP 118/70	
Increased fatigue and feels achy	
Has mild nausea	
Reports tearing in left eye with "gunky stuff," is itchy and uncomfortable	
Takes vitamins and "very rarely needs to use an inhaler"	

2. NGN Item Type: Drop-Down Cloze

19.1.2 Choose the *most likely* options for the information missing from the statement below by selecting from the list of options provided.

Based on the client's assessment data, the findings of T 101.8°F (38.8°C), pleuritic pain, and crackles may indicate _____1_____. The client's "gunky" and uncomfortable eye may be due to _____2_____.

Options for 1	Options for 2
Atelectasis	Allergy
Pneumonia	Sinus infection
Influenza	Conjunctivitis

Scenario

One hour later, the healthcare provider (HCP) has seen the client and writes the following orders:

Health History	Nurses' Notes	Vital Signs	Laboratory Results	**Healthcare Provider Orders**

- Chest x-ray
- WBC
- Sputum C & S
- O₂ prn to keep O₂ saturation above 92%
- Levoflaxacin 750 mg IV daily
- Trimethoprim/polymyxin B eye drops, 1 drop every 3 to 4 hours left eye
- Admit to medical unit

1. NGN Item Type: Multiple Response Select All That Apply

19.2.1 Based on the patient's current treatment plan, the patient's priority outcomes will be to accomplish which of the following? Select all that apply.

A. Clear lung fields
B. Increase activity tolerance
C. Increase energy
D. Decrease chest pain
E. Improve ventilation
F. Decrease temperature
G. Increase comfort left eye

2. NGN Item Type: Matrix Multiple Choice

19.2.2 Use an X to indicate which actions listed in the left column would be included in the plan of care for this patient.

Nursing Actions	Implementation
Monitor respiratory rate, depth, and ease of respirations	
Reinforce that sputum cultures will be needed every 2 to 4 weeks	
Provide adequate rest	
Relieve pleuritic chest pain	
Provide oxygen as prescribed	
Reinforce cough and deep breath 5 to 10 times per hour while awake	
Reinforce teaching of home oxygen	
Increase fluid intake	
Assist Registered Nurse as needed to administer IV antibiotics	
Prepare for mechanical ventilation	

Scenario

Two days later, the client is preparing to go home the following day. Supplemental oxygen has not been needed and the client's cough has decreased. The client will go home on the oral antibiotic doxycycline. Current vital signs are T 99.4°F (37.4°C), P 82, R 16, BP 116/72. The client asks the nurse how to avoid getting pneumonia again.

1. NGN Item Type: Multiple Response Select All That Apply

19.3.1 When providing discharge teaching, the practical nursing student reinforces which of the following information? Select all that apply.
   A. Continue the increased fluid intake
   B. Stop taking the eye drops as soon as the eye starts to feel better
   C. Decrease exposure to people with respiratory infections
   D. Notify your primary health care provider of an increase in symptoms such as fever or dyspnea
   E. Get the pneumococcal vaccine
   F. Adhere to the 4 weeks of home antibiotics
   G. Importance of methods of hand washing

Scenario

The following day, the client is ready to go home. LVN assists the client to pack up their things and then documents in the client's chart.

Health History	Nurses' Notes	Vital Signs	Laboratory Results	Healthcare Provider Orders

1345: Client states, "I'm glad to know that I can help stay well. I will wash my hands with soap and water." Client has been able to ambulate in the hallway without dyspnea and has a decreased cough and sputum production. Client states they are still having pleuritic chest pain. Client's lungs sounds are diminished in the bases with no crackles heard. Client states, "I will be resting at home a lot the next week, and then I will be cutting back at work to a much more normal level. I also know I will need to finish all my antibiotics at home. But I'm not going to get the pneumococcal vaccine." T 99.4°F (37.4°C). Left eye less red without discharge noted.

1. NGN Item Type: Highlight Text

19.4.1 Highlight the findings that indicate the patient is progressing as expected.

Health History	Nurses' Notes	Vital Signs	Laboratory Results	Healthcare Provider Orders

1345: Client states, "I'm glad to know that I can help stay well. I will wash my hands with soap and water." Client has been able to ambulate in the hallway without dyspnea and has a decreased cough and sputum production. Client states they are still having pleuritic chest pain. Client's lungs sounds are diminished in the bases with no crackles heard. Client states, "I will be resting at home a lot the next week, and then I will be cutting back at work to a much more normal level. I also know I will need to finish all my antibiotics at home. But I'm not going to get the pneumococcal vaccine." T 99.4°F (37.4°C). Left eye less red without discharge noted.

Outcome

The student will be able to integrate clinical judgment in assessing, planning, implementing, and evaluating care of the client with a thyroid disorder.

Scenario

A 68-year-old client was brought into a clinic by their daughter. The client lives alone and their daughter lives in a nearby state and visits every few weeks. The daughter states she's seen some changes in her parent in the last couple of months and is worried about dementia. The client is taken to a room by the practical nurse to gather initial information and documents in the chart.

Health History	Nurses' Notes	Healthcare Provider Orders	Laboratory Results

Vital Signs	1045
Temperature (F/C)	96.7°/35.9°
Heart Rate (bpm)	62
Respirations (bpm)	16
Blood Pressure (mmHg)	106/58

Nurses' Notes

1045: Client comes to clinic accompanied by daughter who states has seen recent changes in health and behavior. Client has a history of osteoarthritis. Daughter states is "not sure if parent is confused or forgetful" and reports they haven't "been going to women's group at church." Daughter states parent makes excuses not to do things and says they can't, and usually likes to garden and read. Client reports stiff knees and states "I'm liking the heat up to 80 degrees inside right now." Client also reports weight gain of 20 lbs over recent months. States, "I haven't had a bowel movement in a couple of days, which has become more usual recently." Noted clear lung sounds, S1S2, bowel sounds hypoactive, cool, puffy, dry skin, client wearing glasses.

1. NGN Item Type: Highlight Text

20.1.1 Highlight the assessment findings that require follow-up by the nurse.

Health History	Nurses' Notes	Healthcare Provider Orders	Laboratory Results

Vital Signs	1045
Temperature (F/C)	96.7°/35.9°
Heart Rate (bpm)	62
Respirations (bpm)	16
Blood Pressure (mmHg)	106/58

Nurses' Notes

1045: Client comes to clinic accompanied by daughter who states has seen recent changes in health and behavior. Client has a history of osteoarthritis. Daughter states is "not sure if parent is confused or forgetful" and reports they haven't "been going to women's group at church." Daughter states parent makes excuses not to do things and says they can't, and usually likes to garden and read. Client reports stiff knees and states, "I'm liking the heat up to 80 degrees inside right now." Client also reports weight gain of 20 lbs over recent months. States, "I haven't had a bowel movement in a couple of days, which has become more usual recently." Noted clear lung sounds, S1S2, bowel sounds hypoactive, cool, puffy, dry skin, client wearing glasses.

2. NGN Item Type: Multiple Response Select All That Apply

20.1.2 Which nursing assessment findings support the patient's probable diagnosis of hypothyroidism? Select all that apply.

A. VS: T 96.7°F (35.9°C), P 62, R 16, BP 106/58

B. Daughter states she's "not sure if parent is confused or forgetful

C. Weight gain 20 lbs

D. Cool, puffy, dry skin, bowel sounds hypoactive

E. Reports "haven't had a bowel movement in a couple of days, which has become more usual recently"

F. Reports "hasn't been going to women's group at church"

G. Reports "knees are pretty stiff"

H. Daughter states parent "usually likes to garden and read"

I. Reports "I'm liking the heat up to 80 degrees inside right now"

J. Daughter states parent "makes excuses not to do things and says they can't"

Scenario

The client's primary health care provider (PHCP) ordered labs to be drawn and a follow-up visit the following week. At the follow-up appointment, the following data were documented by the practical nursing student:

Health History	Nurses' Notes	Healthcare Provider Orders	Laboratory Results

Vital Signs	1440
Temperature (F/C)	96.1°/35.6°
Heart Rate (bpm)	60
Respirations (bpm)	16
Blood Pressure (mmHg)	102/58

Nurses' Notes

1440: Client returns with daughter for follow-up visit. Daughter reports she's been finding client using a heating pad on high a lot of the day to stay warm. Client reports has had a little nausea and has taken a few Tums (calcium carbonate). Client reports joints seem to be stiffer with more pain. Daughter states, "I'm worried my parent hasn't been taking their arthritis medication."

Health History	Nurses' Notes	Healthcare Provider Orders	Laboratory Results

Lab Test	Client	Normal
T4	**3.8** mcg/dL	5–12 mcg/dL
TSH	**12.1** mU/L	0.4–4 mU/L

1. NGN Item Type: Drop-Down Cloze

20.2.1 Choose the *most likely* options for the information missing from the statement below by selecting from the list of options provided.

Based on the client's current condition, the patient's **priority** need will be to prevent ____1____ .
In addition, they will need interventions to prevent ____2____, ____3____, and ____4____.

Options for 1	Options for 2	Options for 3	Options for 4
Exophthalmos	Weight loss	Further constipation	Social isolation
Myxedema coma	Secondary hyperthyroidism	Hashimoto's thyroiditis	Medication noncompliance
Thyrotoxicosis	Thermal skin injuries	Goiter	Falls

Scenario

The practical nursing student checks the PHCP orders and reviews the plan of care.

Health History	Nurses' Notes	Healthcare Provider Orders	Laboratory Results

Levothyroxine 25 mcg per day by mouth
Follow-up labs in 6 weeks
Return to clinic in 7 weeks

1. NGN Item Type: Matrix Multiple Choice

20.3.1 Use an X for the reinforced nursing teaching listed below that is <u>indicated</u> (appropriate or necessary) or <u>contraindicated</u> (could be harmful) for the client's care at this time. Only one selection can be made for each nursing action.

Nursing Action	Indicated	Contraindicated
Use lotion on skin and massage it in while skin is so dry.		
This condition is from a nodule on your thyroid gland.		
Stay warm with extra clothing and heat inside but be careful of the heating pad.		
Take your thyroid medication every day on an empty stomach and use a medicine box keeper it if helps remembering.		
Your forgetfulness and lack of energy will get better within weeks once you start taking your thyroid medication daily.		
Make sure to eat a high-calorie diet.		
You may need to have the thyroid medication given intravenously.		

Scenario

Seven weeks later, the client and daughter visit the PHCP clinic. The client's daughter asks if the practical nurse can go over again what they need to remember for the thyroid medication.

Health History	Nurses' Notes	Healthcare Provider Orders	Laboratory Results

Vital Signs	0830
Temperature (F/C)	96.1°/35.6°
Heart Rate (bpm)	60
Respirations (bpm)	16
Blood Pressure (mmHg)	102/58

T 97.8°F (36.6°C), P 70, R 16, BP 118/70.

Nurses' Notes
0830: Client returns with daughter for follow-up visit at week 7. The client's weight has dropped by 6 lbs. The daughter states client seems to be so much better, feeling better and remembering things.

Health History	Nurses' Notes	Healthcare Provider Orders	Laboratory Results

Lab Test	Client	Normal
T4	6 mcg/dL	5–12 mcg/dL
TSH	3.9 mU/L	0.4–4 mU/L

1. NGN Item Type: Matrix Multiple Choice

20.4.1 The practical nurse reinforces teaching on the client's levothyroxine. Use an X to indicate which actions listed in the left column would be included in the plan of care for this patient.

Nursing Actions	Implementation
Take the levothyroxine on a full stomach.	
Take the levothyroxine at the same time every morning.	
Do not stop taking the levothyroxine without the PHCP orders.	
It can be expensive to take these medications, so it's OK to switch from brand name to generic.	
It is OK to take the levothyroxine with your Tums (calcium carbonate).	
Report any symptoms getting worse again such as your low temperature and lethargy.	
Report any symptoms of too much of the medication such as tremors, palpitations, diarrhea, or insomnia.	
Make sure to take your levothyroxine with water and not coffee or other beverages.	

2. NGN Item Type: Matrix Multiple Choice

20.4.2 At the follow-up appointment, the nurse assesses the following statements made by the client. Use an X next to the findings that indicate successful outcomes.

Patient Statement	Successful Outcomes
"I will take my levothyroxine every morning at 7 am with water and will have breakfast at 8 am."	
"I have turned down the temperature in my house because I'm not so cold anymore."	
"I use my medicine keeper box to keep me on track."	
"Now that I feel better, I won't need my thyroid levels checked again."	
"My knees are still pretty stiff."	
"My women's group at church is so happy that I have the energy to be there again."	
"Did you see my weight? I've lost 6 pounds already!"	

21

Urinary Tract Infection

Outcome

The student will demonstrate knowledge of clinical judgment and evidence-based treatment for clients with a urinary tract infection.

Scenario

A 62-year-old client is admitted for a left knee replacement. The LPN arrives for their shift the second postop day and completes a morning assessment.

Health History	Nurses' Notes	Healthcare Provider Orders	Laboratory Results

A 62-year-old client has a history of severe osteoarthritis to both hands and knees and is admitted for a left knee replacement. Medications include celecoxib (on hold preoperatively), ibuprofen (on hold preoperatively), and vitamins.

Health History	Nurses' Notes	Healthcare Provider Orders	Laboratory Results

Day 2

Vital Signs	0745
Temperature (F/C)	101.1°/38.4 °
Heart Rate (bpm)	96
Respirations (bpm)	18
Blood Pressure (mmHg)	126/76
Oxygen saturation	96% on room air
Height	5'5"
Weight	182 lb
BMI	30.3

Nurses' Notes

0745: Client is recovering well from surgery, at 24 hours postoperatively had indwelling catheter discontinued. Client has been up ambulating with physical therapy and is anticipating discharge on the third postop day. Client taking Norco prn for postop left knee pain. Client reports has been helped to the BSC three times in the past several hours with frequency and urgency. States having lower abdominal discomfort. Denies chest pain, shortness of breath, or cough. Knee pain is currently 3/10 on a 0 to 10 pain scale. Left knee dressing is clean, dry, and intact. Assisted client to the BSC and emptied 100 mL of cloudy, foul-smelling urine.

Health History	Nurses' Notes	Healthcare Provider Orders	Laboratory Results

Lab Test	Client	Normal
White blood cell count	WBC **11,450** mm^3	4.5 to 11.0 mm^3

1. NGN Item Type: Highlighting/Enhanced Hot Spot

21.1.1 Highlight the assessment findings that require follow-up by the LPN.

Health History	Nurses' Notes	Healthcare Provider Orders	Laboratory Results

A 62-year-old client has a history of severe osteoarthritis to both hands and knees and is admitted for a left knee replacement. Medications include celecoxib (on hold preoperatively), ibuprofen (on hold preoperatively), and vitamins.

Health History	Nurses' Notes	Healthcare Provider Orders	Laboratory Results

Day 2

Vital Signs	**0745**
Temperature (F/C)	101.1°/38.4°
Heart Rate (bpm)	96
Respirations (bpm)	18
Blood Pressure (mmHg)	126/76
Oxygen saturation	96% on room air
Height	5'5"
Weight	182 lb
BMI	30.3

Nurses' Notes

0745: Client is recovering well from surgery, at 24 hours postoperatively had indwelling catheter discontinued. Client has been up ambulating with physical therapy and is anticipating discharge on the third postop day. Client taking Norco prn for postop left knee pain. Client reports has been helped to the BSC three times in the past several hours with frequency and urgency. States having lower abdominal discomfort. Denies chest pain, shortness of breath, or cough. Knee pain is currently 3/10 on a 0 to 10 pain scale. Left knee dressing is clean, dry, and intact. Assisted client to the BSC and emptied 100 mL of cloudy, foul-smelling urine.

Health History	Nurses' Notes	Healthcare Provider Orders	Laboratory Results

Lab Test	Client	Normal
White blood cell count	WBC **11,450** mm³	4.5 to 11.0 mm³

2. NGN Item Type: Drop-Down Cloze

21.1.2 Choose the *most likely* options for the information missing from the statement below by selecting from the list of options provided.

Based on the client's assessment data, the LPN determines the findings may be due to ____1____, which is most likely caused by ____2____.

Indications for 1	Indications for 2
Incisional infection	Obesity
Urinary tract infection	Limited mobility
Surgical pain	Indwelling catheter

Scenario

One hour later, the NP has been notified and the LPN receives new orders.

Health History	Nurses' Notes	Healthcare Provider Orders	Laboratory Results

Day 2

Urine culture and sensitivity now

Trimethoprim/sulfamethoxazole double strength (160 mg/800 mg) one po Q 12 hours

Phenazopyridine hydrochloride 200 mg one po TID

1. NGN Item Type: Multiple Response Select N

21.2.1 **When planning care for this client, for which three priority potential complications would the LPN monitor? Select all that apply.**
   A. Deep vein thrombosis
   B. Urosepsis
   C. Pneumonia
   D. Septic shock
   E. Pyelonephritis
   F. Stress ulcer

2. NGN Item Type: Matrix Multiple Choice

21.2.2 **Use an X for the nursing actions listed below that are <u>indicated</u> (appropriate or necessary) or <u>contraindicated</u> (could be harmful) for the client's care at this time. Only one selection can be made for each nursing action.**

Nursing Action	Indicated	Contraindicated
Collect urine cultures every 12 hours		
Place client on contact precautions		
Assist with administration of prescribed medications		
Provide heat to the abdomen		
Use sterile technique when inserting urinary catheter if prescribed		
Encourage client to increase fluids to as much as 3,000 mL per day		

Scenario

The next morning, the LPN is reassessing the client and discussing the client's discharge home later that afternoon.

Health History	Nurses' Notes	Healthcare Provider Orders	Laboratory Results

Day 3

Vital Signs	**0745**
Temperature (F/C)	98.0°/36.7°
Heart Rate (bpm)	82
Respirations (bpm)	18
Blood Pressure (mmHg)	128/78
Oxygen saturation	96% on room air
Height	5'5"
Weight	180 lb
BMI	30.3

Nurses' Notes

0745: Client is recovering well, anticipating discharge this afternoon. Client reports frequency and urgency when urinating is "almost gone" and has continued lower abdominal discomfort. Knee pain reported at 2/10. Reinforced client will need to take medications for UTI as prescribed. Reminded client to void every 2 to 3 hours and continue to increase fluid intake.

Health History	Nurses' Notes	Healthcare Provider Orders	Laboratory Results

Lab Test	Client	Normal
White blood cell count	WBC 9,626 mm³	4.5 to 11.0 mm³

1. NGN Item Type: Multiple Response Select All That Apply

21.3.1 What other health teaching should the nurse include in reinforcing teaching regarding trimethoprim/sulfamethoxazole and phenazopyridine hydrochloride at this time? Select all that apply.

    A. Take the antibiotic on an empty stomach with a full glass of water.

    B. Take your antibiotic at evenly spaced times during the day.

    C. Get out in the sunlight, it will be a good source of vitamin D for your healing knee.

    D. Take the phenazopyridine hydrochloride for the entire course of the antibiotics.

    E. Continue to take the antibiotic until the prescribed amount is finished.

    F. Urine may turn a blue or blue-green color that may stain your clothing.

2. NGN Item Type: Matrix Multiple Choice

21.3.2 For each assessment finding, use an X to indicate whether the interventions were <u>effective</u> (helped to meet expected outcomes), <u>ineffective</u> (did not help to meet expected outcomes), or <u>unrelated</u> (not related to the expected outcomes). Each row must have only one option selected.

Assessment Finding	Effective	Ineffective	Unrelated
Client reports frequency and urgency when urinating is "almost gone"			
Weight 180 lbs			
Knee pain is reported at 2/10			
WBC 9,626 mm³			
T 98.0°F (36.7°C)			
Client reports continued lower abdominal discomfort			

22

SECTION 3 MATERNITY

Prenatal Care

Outcome

The learner will correctly identify required actions to manage a client with prenatal care needs.

SLO/Objective

Organize and interpret client information to demonstrate understanding of adaptations to first trimester pregnancy.

Scenario

The LPN working in an OB/GYN clinic takes a client to an exam room and documents in the chart.

Health History	Nurses' Notes	Vital Signs	Laboratory Results

J.S. is a 30-year-old new client presenting to the OB/GYN clinic with a positive pregnancy test. This client has had regular menses since age 13 and her current menstrual period is 3 weeks late. J.S. has a supportive partner and they have been trying to conceive their first pregnancy for 8 months.

Health History	Nurses' Notes	Vital Signs	Laboratory Results

The practical nurse compiles the following client information from the clinic intake form:
- Reports nausea
- Client reports breast tenderness
- Presence of quickening
- Abdominal enlargement
- Positive pregnancy test
- Increased urinary frequency
- Ballottement
- Skin pigmentation changes

1. NGN Item Type: Multiple Response Select All That Apply

22.1.1 Which assessment findings are presumptive of pregnancy? Select all that apply.
  a. Nausea
  b. Amenorrhea
  c. Breast tenderness
  d. Abdominal enlargement
  e. Positive pregnancy test
  f. Increased urinary frequency
  g. Ballottement
  h. Skin pigmentation changes

2. NGN Item Type: Drop-Down Cloze

22.1.2 Choose the *most likely options* for the information missing from the statements below by selecting from the lists of options provided.

The nurse explains to the client that in the first trimester, nausea with or without vomiting is due to _____1_____. Breast tenderness in the first trimester is common and can be attributed to _____2_____. Additional discomforts experienced in the first trimester could include _____3_____.

Options for 1	Options for 2	Options for 3
Increased gastric motility	Increased pigmentation	Headaches
Elevated hormones	Limited vascular supply	Dyspnea
Increased oxygen consumption	Hypertrophy of breast tissue	Round ligament pain
Exchange of nutrients within the placenta	Fluid retention	Urinary frequency

Scenario

The healthcare provider orders an ultrasound.

Health History	Nurses' Notes	Vital Signs	Laboratory Results

The healthcare provider orders an ultrasound. An hour later, the client has the ultrasound performed and the provider confirms pregnancy. The pregnancy is dated as 8 weeks by ultrasound. Following the ultrasound, the client appears worried and verbalizes concerns that the nausea and food aversions may negatively affect the growing fetus.

1. NGN Item Type: Multiple Response Select All That Apply

22.2.1 When planning care for this client in the first trimester, which high-risk complications of severe nausea and vomiting in the first trimester would the nurse alert the client to? Select all that apply.

a. Dehydration
b. Elevated blood pressure
c. Increased blood glucose levels
d. Increased risk for infection
e. Electrolyte imbalance
f. Risk for imbalanced nutrition
g. Decreased urination
h. Depression
i. Miscarriage
j. Hospitalization

2. NGN Item Type: Matrix Multiple Choice

22.2.2 The nurse discusses strategies with the client to incorporate nutritional foods into the daily diet and suggestions for battling nausea in the first trimester. Which of the following are helpful strategies? Use an X to indicate which intervention the nurse identifies in the health teaching as indicated or contraindicated.

Health Teaching	Indicated	Contraindicated
Eating small meals frequently can help with nausea		
Unpasteurized food can be consumed in small amounts		
Daily iron supplementation is recommended with pregnancy		
Ginger consumption can reduce mild to moderate nausea and vomiting		
Prescribed medication may be indicated if nausea and vomiting persist		

Scenario

Health History	Nurses' Notes	Vital Signs	Laboratory Results

The client verbalizes excitement with the confirmation of the pregnancy. J.M. mentions that even with experiencing pregnancy symptoms, the pregnancy does not feel "quite real." Psychosocial adaptations to pregnancy are discussed with client.

1. NGN Item Type: Drop-Down Cloze

22.3.1 Choose the *most likely* options for the information missing from the statements below by selecting from the lists of options provided.

Based on the understanding of psychosocial changes that occur with pregnancy, the nurse explains that _____1_____ is a common feeling for women in the first trimester. As the pregnancy progresses and becomes visually apparent, many women experience changes in _____2_____. In the third trimester, _____3_____ signify increased vulnerability and dependence on the partner.

Options for 1	Options for 2	Options for 3
Fear	Mood	Diet changes
Ambivalence	Independence	Reflection
Disappointment	Gender roles	Mood swings
Acceptance	Body image	Sleep habits

Scenario

Twenty minutes later the practical nurse closes the visit asking the client if there are any questions about today's visit and documents in the chart.

Health History	Nurses' Notes	Vital Signs	Laboratory Results

The practical nurse asks the client if there are any questions about today's visit. The client denies having any further questions and verbalizes understanding about the information discussed at the clinic. A follow-up prenatal visit is scheduled in 4 weeks.

1. NGN Item Type: Multiple Response Select All That Apply

22.4.1 Which statements demonstrate effective client teaching? Select all that apply.
   a. "Small, frequent meals should help with my nausea."
   b. "I know my nausea is caused by a decrease in hormone levels."
   c. "Urinary frequency is common and expected in the first trimester."
   d. "I need to take an iron supplement in addition to my prenatal vitamin."
   e. "I can try eating products with ginger listed as an ingredient to help with constipation."
   f. "I will let my provider know if I am not able to keep fluid or fluids down."
   g. "Even though I don't feel very attached to this pregnancy yet, this is not an uncommon feeling in the first trimester."
   h. "Today my pregnancy was confirmed by ultrasound."

23

Labor

Outcome

The learner will correctly assess client progression through labor to delivery, apply concepts and appropriate nursing interventions to facilitate patient-centered and family-focused care.

Scenario

An LPN working on a labor unit admits a new client and documents in the chart.

Health History	Nurses' Notes	Vital Signs	Laboratory Results

0900:

Client presents to labor and delivery for evaluation of labor, reporting being 39 weeks pregnant with her first child. About 2 hours ago, the client was awakened by irregular contractions and, when getting into the shower, felt a "large gush of fluid." The client then called the obstetric provider, who recommended coming to the hospital labor unit for further evaluation.

0915:

The client is taken into the triage area for further evaluation. The admission nurse completes an initial assessment and compiles the following subjective and objective information:

- Continuous leaking of clear fluid from the vagina
- Term pregnancy
- Fetal movement palpated
- No known allergies
- Reports of irregular uterine contractions
- Reports "shortness of breath" after walking up flight of stairs
- Client has a birth plan
- Support person is at the bedside

1. NGN Item Type: Multiple Response Select All That Apply

23.1.1 The practical nurse reviews the admission note. Which assessment findings require follow-up by the nurse? Select all that apply.

A. Continuous leaking of clear fluid from the vagina

B. Term pregnancy

C. Fetal movement palpated

D. No known allergies

E. Reports of irregular uterine contractions

F. Reports "shortness of breath" after walking up a flight of stairs

G. Client has a birth plan

H. Support person is at the bedside

2. NGN Item Type: Drop-Down Cloze

23.1.2 Choose the *most likely* options for the information missing from the statements below by selecting from the lists of options provided.

Based on the client's assessment data, the nurse remembers _____1_____ could be a sign of latent labor. Latent labor could be occurring due to _____2_____. The client report of _____3_____ in latent labor is a reassuring sign.

Options for 1	Options for 2	Options for 3
Shortness of breath	Continuous leaking of clear fluid from the vagina	No known allergies
Term pregnancy	Fetal movement	A birth plan
Abdominal cramping	Shortness of breath	Fetal movement
Fetal movement	Term pregnancy	Shortness of breath

Scenario

Health History	Nurses' Notes	Vital Signs	Laboratory Results

0945:
Client's membranes determined to be spontaneously ruptured with positive nitrazine paper test and visual pooling of fluid. The client verbalizes desire for labor to progress. Reports contractions becoming more regular in frequency and stronger.

0950:
The obstetric provider is updated on client status, orders received for admission to labor and delivery. The client is moved from the triage area into a labor and delivery room.

Health History	Nurses' Notes	Vital Signs	Laboratory Results	Healthcare Provider Orders

0950:
Admission of term pregnancy to labor and delivery following spontaneous rupture of membranes. Vital signs Q hour. Intermittent external fetal and contraction monitoring 20 minutes every hour. Encourage ambulation and upright labor positions. Limit sterile cervical exams. Place peripheral saline lock for intravenous access.

1. NGN Item Type: Multiple Response Select All That Apply

23.2.1 When planning care for the client with a term pregnancy and spontaneous rupture of membranes, which potential complications should the nurse be aware of? Select all that apply.

A. Nausea and vomiting

B. Increased risk for infection

C. Umbilical cord prolapse

D. Fetal heart rate decelerations

E. Labor dystocia

F. Oligohydramnios

G. Fetal lung maturity

H. Fetal tachycardia

2. NGN Item Type: Multiple Response Select All That Apply

23.2.2 **When reinforcing client teaching regarding the use of external fetal surveillance and contraction monitoring during labor, which of the following information would be important for the nurse to include? Select all that apply.**

   A. It is important to monitor the fetus during labor.
   B. In the active phase of labor, fetal heart rate monitoring will occur every 2 hours.
   C. If analgesia is given in labor, we will continuously monitor the fetal heart rate.
   D. Fetal heart rate monitoring assesses oxygenation of the fetus during labor.
   E. Fetal heart rate patterns can be diagnostic if complications arise in labor.
   F. The obstetric provider will determine what is a normal fetal heart rate pattern.
   G. Contraction patterns can influence fetal oxygen supply.
   H. In some instances, an internal fetal surveillance and contraction monitor may be placed since the membranes have ruptured.

Scenario

As the client progresses the LPN documents in the client's chart.

Health History	**Nurses' Notes**	Vital Signs	Laboratory Results

1600:
The client has regular contractions every 2 minutes. Is progressing through active labor with a supportive family member at bedside. The client has frequently requested nurse assistance for position changes. The client has also utilized breathing techniques during contractions and reports feeling an increase of pressure in the perineum and a strong desire to push. Provider is updated on client status with orders received.

Health History	Nurses' Notes	**Vital Signs**	Laboratory Results

1600:
Vital signs: temperature 98.6°F (37°C), pulse 75 beats per minute, respirations 22 breaths per minutes, pulse oximetry (SpO_2) 95% on room air, blood pressure 126/60 mmHg. Fetal heart rate: 145 with accelerations and variability, category 1 tracing. Contractions every 2 minutes lasting 65 seconds.

Health History	Nurses' Notes	Vital Signs	Laboratory Results	**Healthcare Provider Orders**

1605:
Nurse to verify cervical dilation with sterile vaginal exam. If the client's cervix is fully dilated, and client is feeling the urge to push, the nurse may begin instructing and assisting the client in pushing efforts.

1. NGN Item Type: Drop-Down Rationale

23.3.1 Choose the *most likely options* for the information missing from the statement by selecting from the lists of options provided.

In the second stage of labor, the nurse would _____1_____ because _____2_____.

Options for 1	Options for 2
Advise client the time spent pushing in the second stage of labor is 2 hours	Allowing time for the perineum to stretch will minimize tearing and tissue trauma
Position the client in a modified squatting position for pushing and delivery	The position of the baby, maternal efforts, and position of mom can influence this
Employ breathing techniques between contractions to expedite the delivery	Maternal positioning can facilitate fetal descent and ease of delivery

2. NGN Item Type: Multiple Response Select N

23.3.2 During the second stage of labor, prior to delivery, the nurse assesses the client's understanding from the following statements. Select the three statements that indicate the clients understanding.

A. "I do not have to be in the lithotomy position for delivery."

B. "If I can control my breathing with pushing, my chances of perineal tearing are decreased."

C. "I should continue to push even if I am not having a contraction."

D. "Fetal monitoring ensures my baby will be okay while pushing."

E. "After delivery, I will need to wait to hold my baby."

F. "The placenta will need to be delivered after the baby is born."

Assessment of Newborn

Outcome

Organize and interpret information about a term newborn following vaginal delivery to apply concepts of extrauterine adaptation and appropriate nursing interventions for client-centered care.

Scenario

The LPN is working in the OB Unit and checks and documents in the chart.

Health History	Nurses' Notes	Vital Signs	Laboratory Results

1000: A term infant is born on the labor unit of the local hospital. The infant was delivered following a second labor stage of 1.5 hours, without complications, and was placed immediately skin-to-skin to facilitate transition for the first hour of life.

1001: At 1 minute of age, the newborn has a strong cry, is responsive to being vigorously dried with a towel, has active and spontaneous motion, some presence of acrocyanosis in the extremities, and a heart rate of 155. A 1-minute APGAR score was assigned.

1003: Following a period of delayed cord clamping, the cord was clamped and cut. Assessments and vital signs including temperature continue to be completed with the infant on mother's chest. Delivery personnel remain at the bedside and include the provider, delivery nurse, and LPN. Support for the mother and newborn includes the support person who is at the bedside.

1. NGN Item Type: Multiple Response Select All That Apply

24.1.1 When planning care for the newborn client, which assessments would be prioritized by the RN to obtain an APGAR score? Select all that apply.

A. Responsive to vigorous drying
B. Second stage of labor 1.5 hours
C. Spontaneous motion
D. Strong cry
E. Acrocyanosis
F. Heart rate of 155

2. NGN Item Type: Drag-and-Drop Cloze

24.1.2 Choose the *most likely options* for the information missing from the statements below by selecting from the lists of options provided.

Based on the assessment data, the nurse understands that the purpose of assigning an APGAR score is to _____1_____ the newborn _____2_____ right after delivery.

Options for 1	Options for 2
Evaluate	Gestational age
Diagnose	Gender
Remediate	Condition

Scenario

Health History	Nurses' Notes	Vital Signs	Laboratory Results

1100: After 1 hour of skin-to-skin time and an attempt at breastfeeding, the newborn is brought to the bedside radiant warmer for a full assessment. The LPN completes the vital signs and the assessment with the delivery RN. The height, weight, and head circumference are also measured and documented.

Health History	Nurses' Notes	Vital Signs	Laboratory Results

1100: Newborn vital signs: temperature 98.2°F (36.8°C), pulse 75 beats per minute, respirations 22 breaths per minute, pulse oximetry (SpO$_2$) 95% on room air.

Vital signs: temperature 98.2°F (37°C), pulse 142 beats per minute, respirations 44 breaths per minute, pulse oximetry (SpO$_2$) 95% on room air. Fetal head circumference: 14.1 inches (36 cm), height 19.7 inches (50 cm), weight 7 pounds 7 ounces (3.492 kg).

1. NGN Item Type: Multiple Response Select N

24.2.1 Which three newborn diagnoses are high risk and require additional interventions? Select the three findings that require follow-up.

   A. Neonatal hypoglycemia
   B. Jaundice
   C. Spontaneous ventilation
   D. Effective feeding pattern
   E. Hypothermia
   F. Bowel incontinence

2. NGN Item Type: Matrix Multiple Choice

24.2.2 Which nursing interventions would the LPN anticipate when planning care for the newborn? Use an X to indicate which intervention the nurse identifies as indicated or contraindicated for the newborn plan of care. Each row must have only one response option selected.

Nursing Interventions	Indicated for Plan of Care	Contraindicated for Plan of Care
Promoting skin-to-skin contact		
Assisting with breastfeeding every 4 hours		
Tracking newborn voids and stools		
Monitoring newborn vital signs once a shift		
Giving the newborn a bath 1 hour after delivery		
Administering vitamin K before newborn is 24 hours of age		

Scenario

Health History	Nurses' Notes	Vital Signs	Laboratory Results

Day 2 of hospital stay. 24 hours after delivery.

1000: LPN at bedside for vital sign check and preparing for newborn discharge home. Mother states, "The newborn is breastfeeding every 2 hours for 20 minutes at each breast." Family also noted the presence of meconium stool with diaper changes and several voids during the night.

Health History	Nurses' Notes	Vital Signs	Laboratory Results

1000: Newborn vital signs: axillary temperature 96.2°F (36.8°C), pulse 132 beats per minute, respirations 36 breaths per minute.

1. NGN Item Type: Multiple Response Select All That Apply

24.3.1 When providing newborn teaching, the nurse includes which of the following information? Select all that apply.
  A. The stomach capacity of the newborn is very small.
  B. The newborn is receiving colostrum while feeding, which has protective antibodies.
  C. The frequency of feedings does not determine when transitional milk will appear.
  D. As the newborn feeds, there will be a decrease in the number of voids.
  E. Meconium stool will change in consistency and color with frequent breastfeeding.

Scenario

24 hours after delivery, the LPN reviews the newborn chart to determine readiness for discharge home.

Health History	Nurses' Notes	Vital Signs	Laboratory Results

- Newborn axillary temperature of 36.8°C (98.2°F)
- Newborn breastfeeding 5 minutes every 4 hours
- Newborn has had two meconium stools
- Newborn has a heart rate of 132 beats per minute
- The newborn skin has a yellowed appearance
- Newborn is swaddled and sleeping in separate sleep space
- Newborn has an active Moro reflex

1. NGN Item Type: Highlight Table

24.4.1 Highlight findings that are reassuring for discharge.

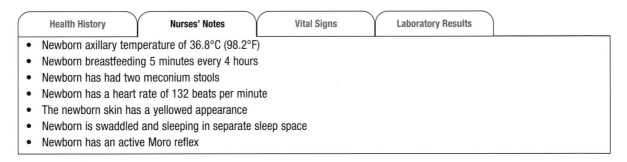

Health History	Nurses' Notes	Vital Signs	Laboratory Results

- Newborn axillary temperature of 36.8°C (98.2°F)
- Newborn breastfeeding 5 minutes every 4 hours
- Newborn has had two meconium stools
- Newborn has a heart rate of 132 beats per minute
- The newborn skin has a yellowed appearance
- Newborn is swaddled and sleeping in separate sleep space
- Newborn has an active Moro reflex

25

Preterm Infant

Outcome

Interpret data obtained by assessment of the preterm infant to organize and apply appropriate nursing care and interventions.

Scenario

A licensed practical nurse is working on the neonatal unit assisting with care of a preterm infant.

Health History	Nurses' Notes	Vital Signs	Laboratory Results

Baby C.A. was born premature at 32 weeks' gestation following a preterm premature rupture of membranes (PPROM), which occurred 36 hours before delivery. Prior to vaginal delivery, the mother received several doses of intravenous antibiotics to prevent infection and two doses of corticosteroids to facilitate fetal lung maturity. Despite attempts to delay preterm delivery with medications, C.A. delivered rapidly after a 30-minute second stage.

Health History	Nurses' Notes	**Vital Signs**	Laboratory Results

Newborn vital signs 5 minutes after delivery: temperature 96.9°F (36.1°C), pulse 120 beats per minute, respiration 64 breaths per minutes, pulse oximetry (SpO$_2$) 90% on room air.

Health History	**Nurses' Notes**	Vital Signs	Laboratory Results

At 5 minutes of age, newborn has acrocyanosis present both extremities bilaterally. One- and 5-minute APGAR scores are 6 and 8. C.A. will be transferred to the neonatal intensive care unit, where transition will continue under specialized care.

APGAR Score	1 Minute	5 Minutes
Activity (muscle tone)	1	2
Pulse	2	2
Grimace (reflex irritability)	1	1
Appearance (skin color)	1	1
Respiration	1	2

1. NGN Item Type: Drop-Down Cloze

25.1.1 Choose the *most likely options* for the information missing from the statements below by selecting from the lists of options provided.

Based on the initial vital signs, the nurse identifies findings requiring immediate follow-up. These include _____1_____ and _____2_____. The nurse understands that these findings along with the maternal history of _____3_____ place the newborn at high risk for _____4_____.

Options for 1	Options for 2	Options for 3	Options for 4
Pulse	Oxygen saturation	Rapid second stage	Congenital anomalies
Temperature	Respiratory rate	Antibiotic administration	Sepsis
Appearance	Activity	PPROM	Hyperthermia

2. NGN Item Type: Multiple Response Select All That Apply

25.1.2 **Which assessment findings are consistent with the delivery of a preterm infant? Select all that apply.**

A. Hypothermia

B. Rapid respiratory rate

C. Fetal lung maturity

D. Oxygen saturation 90% on room air

E. Acrocyanosis

F. Congenital anomalies

Scenario

Health History	Nurses' Notes	Vital Signs	Laboratory Results

C.A. is admitted to the neonatal intensive care unit for close monitoring following preterm delivery, hypothermia, and respiratory rate. A care plan is formulated by the provider to provide individualized and specialized care while on the unit. C.A. is placed on several monitors that continually track and identify changes in vital signs and signal the health care team if they are outside normal parameters.

1. NGN Item Type: Multiple Response Select All That Apply

25.2.1 **Based on the preterm newborn's condition, the LPN anticipates planning care to prevent which of the following four high-risk conditions? Select all that apply.**

A. Sepsis

B. Respiratory distress syndrome

C. Weight gain

D. Retinopathy of prematurity

E. Neural tube defects

F. Club foot

G. Necrotizing enterocolitis

2. NGN Item Type: Matrix Multiple Choice

25.2.2 **The practical nursing student is generating a plan of care for the client for the following nursing actions. Use an X to indicate which interventions are indicated or contraindicated for the plan of care. Each row must only have one response option selected.**

Nursing Action	Indicated	Contraindicated
Provide a neutral thermal environment		
Encourage formula feedings		
Place infant in a supine position		
Maintain a quiet environment		
Encourage parents to touch the newborn		

Scenario

Six weeks later the LPN documents care in the chart.

Health History	Nurses' Notes	Vital Signs	Laboratory Results

6 weeks later: C.A. remains stable in the neonatal intensive care unit following delivery at 32 weeks' gestation. Vital signs are stable, and C.A. has steadily gained weight, progressed to breastfeeding and bottle-feeding breast milk, and is hitting all growth and developmental milestones. The care team meets daily to discuss progress and is working with the family toward a plan for discharge.

1. NGN Item Type: Multiple Response Select All That Apply

25.3.1 When preparing the parents for discharge home with their newborn, which of the following teaching topics will be important to discuss? Select all that apply.
   A. Kangaroo care should not be continued at home.
   B. Follow-up visits with the pediatrician should be prioritized.
   C. Immunizations will need to be delayed until 1 year.
   D. To keep an eye on the newborn, bed sharing is encouraged.
   E. All caregivers should be up to date on vaccinations.
   F. Taking a newborn cardiopulmonary resuscitation (CPR) class is recommended.

2. NGN Item Type: Multiple Response Select All That Apply

25.3.2 Prior to discharge, the LPN reviews the chart of the newborn client. Which findings indicate successful care outcomes? Select all that apply.
   A. Newborn has had no apneic periods for 7 days.
   B. Newborn is breastfeeding on demand and being supplemented as needed with breastmilk.
   C. A pacifier is used to soothe the newborn.
   D. Newborn startle reflex is no longer present.
   E. Newborn has decreased reflux with feedings.
   F. Newborn uses accessory muscles with respirations.

26

Postpartum/Mood Disorder

Outcome

Organize and interpret client information to provide nursing interventions and evaluate the care of the postpartum client.

Scenario

A LVN is working in an obstetric clinic and takes a 28-year-old client to an exam room and documents in the chart.

Health History	Nurses' Notes	Vital Signs	Laboratory Results

J.M. is a 28-year-old client who delivered by cesarean section 4 weeks ago. Following the cesarean section, J.M. stayed in the hospital for 72 hours and then was discharged home with the newborn. J.M. is being seen today in the obstetric clinic for a postsurgical follow-up appointment. It will be the first visit since discharge. While completing the client intake form, the client notes having "a lot of emotions" in the first week after discharge and now reports having trouble sleeping and increased anxiety around caring for the newborn. J.M. describes concern with breastfeeding and is unsure and anxious if the infant is receiving enough breastmilk.

Health History	Nurses' Notes	Vital Signs	Laboratory Results

The intake nurse and practical nurse compile the following information from the patient:
- Four weeks postpartum
- History of cesarean section
- A lot of emotions
- Trouble sleeping
- Increased anxiety
- Disturbed appetite
- Breastfeeding every 2 to 3 hours

1. NGN Item Type: Multiple Response Select N

26.1.1 Which findings require immediate follow-up at a first postsurgical postpartum visit? Select the four findings that require follow-up.

A. Four weeks postpartum
B. A lot of emotions
C. History of cesarean section
D. Trouble sleeping
E. Increased anxiety
F. Disturbed appetite
G. Breastfeeding every 2 to 3 hours

2. NGN Item Type: Matrix Multiple Response

26.1.2 Use an X to specify if the assessment finding is associated with baby blues or postpartum depression. Each row must have at least one response option selected.

Assessment Finding	Baby Blues	Postpartum Depression
Trouble sleeping		
Disturbed appetite		
A lot of emotions		
Increased anxiety		

Scenario

Health History	Nurses' Notes	Vital Signs	Laboratory Results

The nurse inquires if the symptoms the client reports are interfering with the ability to care for the newborn. Client nods in agreement and describes, "I feel inadequate and unsure if I can be a good mother, I am exhausted all the time."

1. NGN Item Type: Drop-Down Rationale

26.2.1 Choose the *most likely options* for the information missing from the statement by selecting from the lists of options provided.

While planning care for this client, the practical nurse knows that this postpartum client is at highest risk for _____1_____ as evidenced by _____2_____.

Options for 1	Options for 2
Mania	Feelings of inadequacy
Bipolar disorder	Mania
Hyperactivity	Psychosis
Self-harm	Feelings of invulnerability

2. NGN Item Type: Matrix Multiple Choice

26.2.2 The practical nurse is working with the RN to generate a plan of care for the client. For each nursing action, use an X to indicate which nursing action is indicated or contraindicated for the client plan of care at this time.

Nursing Action	Indicated	Contraindicated
Diagnose the client's feelings		
Observe for signs and symptoms of strained coping mechanisms		
Promote behaviors that can increase mental health		
Remind the client these feelings are transient and will often go away without treatment		
Provide a list of community mental health support services		

Scenario

Health History	Nurses' Notes	Vital Signs	Laboratory Results

One hour later: The provider has spent ample time with the client exploring symptoms and how they have affected J.M.'s ability to transition into the new parent role. Provider recommends additional treatments that include outpatient psychotherapy and the initiation of antidepressants, discusses signs of worsening anxiety and depression to watch for, and has the client list family or friends to call when feeling overwhelmed. Client verbalizes great relief with the outcome of this visit and states, "I am hopeful that I will be feeling more like myself soon."

1. NGN Item Type: Multiple Response Select All That Apply

26.3.1 The practical nurse is reinforcing provider teaching to the client. Which of the following information should this include? Select all that apply.

A. Communicate if you are feeling hopeless or feel unable to cope.

B. If you feel overwhelmed while caring for your newborn, place the infant in a safe sleep space, walk away, and call a support person for help.

C. Your emotions and feelings will get worse before they begin to get better.

D. Talking to a therapist may help resolve depression and anxiety.

E. When taking medication for depression and anxiety, it is okay to stop taking the medications when you start feeling better.

F. Postpartum depression is an illness that can be treated.

G. You should not be left alone with your baby.

2. NGN Item Type: Multiple Response Select All That Apply

26.3.2 Prior to leaving the clinic, the nurse assesses the client's understanding of the plan of care. Which statements support client understanding? Select all that apply.

A. Client states she will call a family member if she is alone and feeling overwhelmed.

B. Client acknowledges her symptoms are not consistent with postpartum depression.

C. Client verbalizes her intent to follow up with therapist next month.

D. The client states she will follow up with community support services for new moms.

E. The client acknowledges the importance of family and friend support during this transition.

27

Respiratory Syncytial Virus (RSV)

Outcome

Organize care in a manner which provides a complete, age-appropriate/developmentally specific pediatric assessment for a child with respiratory syncytial virus.

Scenario

The LPN has assumed care of a 20-month-old with a diagnosis of respiratory syncytial virus (RSV) admitted to the pediatric floor from the emergency department.

Health History	Nurses' Notes	Vital Signs	Laboratory Results

0900: Client placed in a semi-private room on contact precautions. The client's eyes are closed with a damp washcloth on their forehead, a popsicle is on the bedside table in a cup. The client has frequent coughing and sneezing episodes, with shallow and rapid breathing. Parents appear worried and are at the bedside.

Health History	Nurses' Notes	Vital Signs	Laboratory Results

0900: Vital signs: tympanic temperature 101.2°F (39.4°C), pulse 110 beats per minute, respirations 48 breaths per minute nasal flaring present, blood pressure 95/60, pulse oximetry 90% on 1.5 L humidified oxygen via nasal canula. Pain rating 2/10 using FACES pain scale.

Health History	Nurses' Notes	Vital Signs	Laboratory Results	Healthcare Provider Orders

0905: Inpatient pediatric status. Strict intake and output monitoring, humidified oxygen via nasal cannula, titrate flow to maintain 90% to 95% saturation. Respiratory therapy breathing treatments twice a day. Antipyretic, antiviral medication and intravenous fluids can be administered if patient condition dictates, call for further orders.

1. NGN Item Type: Highlight Table

27.1.1 Highlight the objective assessment findings that would require immediate follow-up.

Health History	Nurses' Notes	Vital Signs	Laboratory Results

0900: Client placed in a semi-private room on contact precautions. The client's eyes are closed with a damp washcloth on their forehead, a popsicle is on the bedside table in a cup. The client has frequent coughing and sneezing episodes, with shallow and rapid breathing. Parents appear worried and are at the bedside.

Health History	Nurses' Notes	Vital Signs	Laboratory Results

0900: Vital signs: tympanic temperature 101.2°F (39.4°C), pulse 110 beats per minute, respirations 48 breaths per minute nasal flaring present, blood pressure 95/60, pulse oximetry 90% on 1.5 L humidified oxygen via nasal canula. Pain rating 2/10 using FACES pain scale.

Health History	Nurses' Notes	Vital Signs	Laboratory Results	Healthcare Provider Orders

0905: Inpatient pediatric status. Strict intake and output monitoring, humidified oxygen via nasal cannula, titrate flow to maintain 90% to 95% saturation. Respiratory therapy breathing treatments twice a day. Antipyretic, antiviral medication and intravenous fluids can be administered if patient condition dictates, call for further orders.

2. NGN Item Type: Multiple Choice Select All That Apply

27.1.2 A nursing student asks the LPN which one of the following assessment findings in a pediatric client with RSV dictates the use of contact precautions? Select all that apply.

A. Temperature of 101.2°F tympanic
B. Frequent coughing and sneezing
C. Use of continuous humidified oxygen
D. Worried family at the bedside
E. Frequent respiratory therapy treatments
F. Respirations of 48

Scenario

Client is moved to a private room on the pediatric unit with continued contact precautions.

Health History	Nurses' Notes	Vital Signs	Laboratory Results

1200: The client appears restless and is crying. Family at the bedsides states the client has not had any wet diapers and is acting tired and hungry but doesn't want to eat a popsicle or drink any fluids. Encouragement given to the parents to keep trying to encourage oral fluids and to not dispose of any soiled diapers.

Health History	Nurses' Notes	Vital Signs	Laboratory Results

1200 Vital signs: tympanic temperature 101.8°F (38.7°C), pulse 115 beats per minute, respirations 44 breaths per minute, blood pressure 93/60, pulse oximetry 90% on 1.5 L humidified oxygen via nasal canula. Pain rating 6/10 using FACES pain scale.

1. NGN Item Type: Drag-and-Drop Rationale

27.2.1 Choose the *most likely options* for the information missing from the statement by selecting from the lists of options provided.

The pediatric client is at high risk for developing _____1_____ as evidenced by _____2_____.

Options for 1	Options for 2
Incontinence	Humidified oxygen
Impaired skin integrity	Decreased oral intake
Dehydration	No voids since admission

2. NGN Item Type: Matrix Multiple Choice

27.2.2 **The LPN and the RN are formulating a plan of care based on the client diagnosis of RSV. Use an X to indicate which of the following nursing actions listed are indicated or contraindicated for the client's care at this time. Each row must have only one response option selected.**

Nursing Actions	Indicated	Contraindicated
Increase humidified oxygen to 4 liters nasal canula		
Record a daily weight		
Implementation of fever-reducing measures		
Evaluate pain using appropriate pain scale every shift		
Document the intake and output of the client every hour		

Scenario

An hour later, the LPN checks in on the client and family and records vital signs.

Health History	**Nurses' Notes**	Vital Signs	Laboratory Results

1300: The pediatric client is awake but tired and watching cartoons and has just finished a popsicle. Family member states they have changed a wet diaper and put it aside.

Health History	Nurses' Notes	**Vital Signs**	Laboratory Results

1300 Vital signs: tympanic temperature 101.8°F (38.7°C), pulse 115 beats per minute, respirations 40 breaths per minute, blood pressure 90/55, pulse oximetry 92% on 1.5 L humidified oxygen via nasal canula. Pain rating 1/10 using FACES pain scale.

1. NGN Item Type: Multiple Response Select All That Apply

27.3.1 **Which nursing actions would be included in a strict intake and output assessment of a pediatric client with RSV? Select all that apply.**
- A. Record every client void on report sheet.
- B. Bowel movements do not need to be included in output measurements.
- C. Use scale at the nurse's station to weigh diaper.
- D. Perform skin turgor assessment on the abdomen.
- E. Record the color, character, and odor of the urine.
- F. Weigh the child every morning.
- G. Fluids from oral suctioning do not need to be counted as output.
- H. Record in mL the electrolyte popsicle as input.
- I. Assess mucous membranes and for the presence of tears.

2. NGN Item Type: Multiple Response Select All That Apply

27.3.2 **The LPN evaluates the effectiveness of the interventions implemented based on assessments during the shift. Which of the following client findings indicate effectiveness? Select all that apply.**
- A. Oral intake of electrolyte popsicle
- B. Voiding present
- C. Lethargy
- D. Pulse 115 beats per minute
- E. T 101.8°F (38.7°C)
- F. O_2 saturation 92% on 1.5 L humidified nasal canula

28

Epilepsy

Outcome

The student will demonstrate comprehensive application of critical thinking in managing the care of the client with epilepsy disorder.

Scenario

A 10-year-old is brought to the pediatrician's office for an unscheduled checkup. The LVN takes the client and mother to a room and begins to gather data.

Health History	Nurses' Notes	Healthcare Provider Orders	Vital Signs

Client was a full-term baby with a normal delivery.
History of three separate ear infections as a toddler. Positive for strep throat last school year.
Client has been developmentally on task for their age each year.

Health History	Nurses' Notes	Healthcare Provider Orders	Vital Signs

1420: Client's mother states she brought in child who had "an episode" last night, but has been completely fine since. Mother states that client was sleeping and one side of their face twisted to one side, their left arm jerked and stiffened, and then their whole body stiffened. The client is alert and oriented and is happy talking with the nurse. Client is currently 76 lbs, 54 inches.

1. NGN Item Type: Drop-Down Cloze

28.1.1 Choose the *most likely* options for the information missing from the statement below by selecting from the list of options provided.

The assessment findings that require immediate follow-up include _____1_____, _____2_____, _____3_____.

Options for 1	Options for 2	Options for 3
Alert and oriented	Left arm jerked and stiffened	History of strep throat
Ear infections	Developmentally on task	Birth delivery
Face twisted to one side	Weight 76 lbs	Whole body stiffened

2. NGN Item Type: Multiple Response Select All That Apply

28.1.2 What further questions could the LVN ask to gain more information? Select all that apply.
A. "How long did the episode last?"
B. "Does the client often have trouble sleeping?"
C. "What was the client's behavior immediately after the episode?"
D. "Was there any loss of consciousness?"
E. "Does the client drink enough fluids each day?"
F. "Was the client incontinent during or after the episode?"
G. "Has the client lost any weight recently?"

Scenario

The NP performs a full exam and has found no abnormalities and has counseled the mother to take the client to the ED with further episodes. Ten days later, the client has another episode and is driven to the ED by their mother. The client is admitted to the pediatric unit for further workup for suspected seizure disorder.

1. NGN Item Type: Drag-and-Drop Cloze

28.2.1 Choose the *most likely* options for the information missing from the statements below by selecting from the lists of options provided.

Based on the client's condition, the client's current **priority** needs will be to prevent _____1_____ and _____2_____.

Options for 1 and 2
Injury
Embarrassment
Incontinence
Fatigue
Status epilepticus
Triggers

2. NGN Item Type: Multiple Response Grouping

28.2.2 Select the anticipated HCP orders from each of the following categories. (Each category must have at least one response option selected.)

Category	Orders
Diagnostics	☐ MRI of brain
	☐ EKG
	☐ EEG
Medications	☐ Tums one po prn upset stomach
	☐ Phenytoin suspension po 85 mg bid
	☐ Carbamazepine 100 mg po bid
Nursing interventions	☐ Keep side rails up
	☐ Pad sharp/hard objects around the bed
	☐ Give phenytoin with milk
	☐ Monitor for side effects of the medications
	☐ Monitor phenytoin levels every morning

Scenario

Three days later, the client has been diagnosed with epilepsy and treatment has been started. There have been no further seizures. The NP has reviewed home care with the client and both parents. Before the planned discharge tomorrow, the LVN is reinforcing teaching.

1. NGN Item Type: Matrix Multiple Choice

28.3.1 Use an X for nursing actions listed below that are <u>indicated</u> (necessary) or <u>contraindicated</u> (could be harmful). Only one selection can be made for each nursing action.

Nursing Action	Indicated	Contraindicated
No bathing or swimming alone and avoid heights		
Wear a helmet for bicycling or skating		
Wear a medical alert bracelet		
Restrain child during a seizure to prevent injury		
Practice careful and thorough oral care		
Phenytoin can cause hyperactivity		
Use a spoon to hold down the tongue during a seizure		
Take medications the same time every day		
After 2 years the child can be evaluated to wean off medications		
Work with teachers and school nurse for medications and social functioning		

2. NGN Item Type: Multiple Response Select All That Apply

28.3.2 The nurse evaluates the effectiveness of actions. Which of the following findings indicate effectiveness? Select all that apply.
A. Fully controlled seizures
B. Safety measures are in place to prevent injury
C. Mom will do everything for them so client can't get hurt
D. Parents and child state how to avoid anything that might trigger seizures
E. Child reports some blurred vision
F. Mom reports she found an epilepsy support group for children for client

29

Communicable Disease

Outcome

The student will demonstrate comprehensive application of critical thinking in managing the care of the client with a communicable disease.

Scenario

A 19-month-old client is brought to the pediatric clinic by their mother. The mother tells the LPN that she first noticed a "funny spot on their head" yesterday morning; by last night, they were on their chest and back, and this morning the spots are everywhere on their body. The client is crying, has a runny nose, and is scratching everything they can reach. The LPN notes the following information.

Health History	Nurses' Notes	Vital Signs	Laboratory Results

Vital Signs	**1030**
Temperature (F/C)	100.2°/37.8° axillary
Heart Rate (bpm)	105 apical
Respirations (bpm)	26
Blood Pressure (mmHg)	90/52

Health History	Nurses' Notes	Vital Signs	Laboratory Results

1030:
- Lungs clear to auscultation
- Heart sounds regular
- Abdomen soft and nontender
- Scratches on both arms and face
- Child irritable and crying
- Rash with over 500 lesions in all stages, some fluid-filled blisters, others macular or papules, some lesions crusted over
- Mom reports poor oral fluid intake
- Blisters inside oral cavity

1. NGN Item Type: Matrix Multiple Choice

29.1.1 Use an X to indicate which client assessment findings require follow-up by the nurse at this time.

Assessment Finding	Assessment Finding That Requires Follow-Up
VS: T 100.2°F (37.8°C) axillary	
P 105 apical, R 26, BP 90/52	
Lungs clear to auscultation	
Heart sounds regular	
Abdomen soft and nontender	
Scratches on both arms and face	
Child irritable and crying	
Rash with over 500 lesions in all stages	
Mom reports poor oral fluid intake	
Blisters inside oral cavity	

2. NGN Item Type: Multiple Response Select N

29.1.2 Which of the *four* nursing assessment findings support the client's probable diagnosis of varicella (chickenpox)?
- A. Mild fever
- B. Rash with lesions in all stages present at the same time
- C. Scratches on arms and face
- D. Child crying
- E. Lesions on mucous membranes of mouth
- F. Rash first on scalp and trunk followed by rest of the body
- G. P 105 apical, R 26, BP 90/52
- H. Runny nose
- I. Poor oral fluid intake

Scenario

Due to the large number of lesions, including inside the mouth as well as the poor oral intake, the client is admitted to the pediatric unit at the local hospital with the diagnosis of varicella.

1. NGN Item Type: Drag-and-Drop Rationale

29.2.1 Choose the *most likely* option from client finding and priority need to fill in each blank in the following sentence.

Based on the client's _____, the **priority** need will be to provide _____?

Client Finding	Priority Need
Child crying	Removal of scabs
Fever	Aspirin for pain
Poor oral fluid intake	Airborne isolation
Rash with lesions in all stages present at the same time	Relief from shingles

2. NGN Item Type: Matrix Multiple Choice

29.2.2 Use an X to indicate which actions listed in the left column would be included in the plan of care for this patient.

Nursing Actions	Relevant Nursing Actions
Trim the child's fingernails	
Apply calamine lotion prn	
Provide a cool oatmeal bath	
Place in contact precautions as indicated	
Administer acyclovir as ordered	
Provide antimicrobial therapy	

Scenario

Two days later, the client is feeling better and is ready for discharge home. The RN has provided discharge teaching and instructions.

1. NGN Item Type: Drop-Down Cloze

29.3.1 Choose the *most likely* options for the information missing from the statement below by selecting from the list of options provided.

The practical nurse reinforces teaching to the client's parents and includes _____1_____ and _____2_____.

Options for 1	Options for 2
Client can go back to day care once they're home.	It's fine at home to give aspirin.
Once the client goes home, keep them isolated until the vesicles have dried up.	Client can be around their cousin with leukemia once they're at home.
Once home, the scratching won't be a problem.	After discharge home, make sure your child doesn't pick at the skin lesions.

2. NGN Item Type: Multiple Response Select All That Apply

29.3.2 Which of the following findings indicate effectiveness of care? Select all that apply.

A. Parents will encourage fluids with items such as sugar-free popsicles and favorite drinks.

B. No scarring occurs.

C. Mom states she bought a new bottle of pediatric acetaminophen for home use.

D. Urine output is over 30 mL per hour.

E. Mom states she'll keep client especially warm once they get home since they have been so sick.

F. No one else in family contracted chickenpox.

G. Dad states they will talk to pediatrician about the varicella vaccination.

Diabetes Mellitus Type 1

30

Outcome

The student will apply critical thinking to planning care for a client with diabetes mellitus type 1.

Scenario

The client is a 16-year-old whose mother brings them to the ED on a Saturday afternoon after severe nausea and vomiting for 2 days. The LPN settles the client and mother in a room and documents current findings.

Health History	Nurses' Notes	Healthcare Provider Orders	Laboratory Results

Vital Signs	**1300**
Temperature (F/C)	97.2°/36.2°
Heart Rate (bpm)	92
Respirations (bpm)	16
Blood Pressure (mmHg)	110/64
Weight	168 lb

Nurses' Notes

1300: Client's mother reports client had a "pretty nasty viral infection with a sore throat that seemed to last forever about 6 weeks ago." The client reports a headache and new fatigue. Client reports is thirsty all the time, has had nausea and vomiting for 2 days, and is currently nauseated. Mother reports that at the yearly check-up with the pediatrician 4 months ago, the client's weight was 180 lb. By fingerstick, current blood sugar is 460 mg/dL. Heart sounds regular, lungs clear to auscultation, abdomen soft and non-tender, oral mucous membranes dry, old bruise on left lower leg. Client's mother is very agitated, pacing and wringing her hands.

1. NGN Item Type: Highlight Text

30.1.1 Highlight the assessment findings that require immediate follow-up by the nurse.

Health History	Nurses' Notes	Healthcare Provider Orders	Laboratory Results

Vital Signs	**1300**
Temperature (F/C)	97.2°/36.2°
Heart Rate (bpm)	92
Respirations (bpm)	16
Blood Pressure (mmHg)	110/64
Weight	168 lb

Nurses' Notes

1300: Client's mother reports client had a "pretty nasty viral infection with a sore throat that seemed to last forever about 6 weeks ago." The client reports a headache and new fatigue. Client reports is thirsty all the time, has had nausea and vomiting for 2 days, and is currently nauseated. Mother reports that at the yearly check-up with the pediatrician 4 months ago, the client's weight was 180 lb. By fingerstick, current blood sugar is 460 mg/dL. Heart sounds regular, lungs clear to auscultation, abdomen soft and nontender, oral mucous membranes dry, old bruise on left lower leg. Client's mother is very agitated, pacing and wringing her hands.

107

2. NGN Item Type: Drop-Down Cloze

30.1.2 Choose the *most likely* options for the information missing from the statement below by selecting from the list of options provided.

The nurse recognizes that, based on the assessment data and patient's history, the patient is currently at risk for _____1_____, _____2_____, and _____3_____.

Indications for 1	Indications for 2	Indications for 3
Recurrent infections	Fluid overload	Hypoglycemia
Phenylketonuria	Hyperglycemia	Stress ulcer
Social isolation	Constipation	Fever

Scenario

The assigned LPN works with the charge RN to develop an anticipated plan of care for the client.

Health History	Nurses' Notes	**Healthcare Provider Orders**	Laboratory Results

1430: Admit to the pediatric unit

1. NGN Item Type: Matrix Multiple Choice

30.2.1 Use an X to indicate which actions listed in the left column would be anticipated to be included in the plan of care for this patient.

Nursing Actions	Implementation
Assist RN with IV fluid 0.9% NS @ 100 mL/hr	
Monitor urine output	
Check blood sugar levels ac & hs	
Administer insulin as prescribed	
Give extra carbohydrates	
Monitor labs especially K+	

Scenario

The client has been settled in a room on the pediatric unit. Orders were received and implemented by the LPN and RN. The following morning, the client is pacing the floor of their room when the practical nurse walks in.

Health History	**Nurses' Notes**	Healthcare Provider Orders	Vital Signs

Day 2

Vital Signs	0745
Temperature (F/C)	97.4°/36.3°
Heart Rate (bpm)	92
Respirations (bpm)	16
Blood Pressure (mmHg)	118/68

Nurses' Notes

0745: Client states the nausea and vomiting have decreased. Client has had several insulin injections, including the most recent at 0630. IV fluids were discontinued at 0630 by the RN. Client states they don't feel like eating and refusing breakfast. Client states, "Why is this happening to me?" and wants to go home.

1. NGN Item Type: Drop Down Cloze-

30.3.1 Choose the *most likely* options for the information missing from the statements below by selecting from the lists of options provided.

Based on the client's current condition, the client's **priority** need will be to prevent _____1_____ as evidenced by the client's_____2_____, _____2_____, and _____2_____.

Options for 1	Options for 2
Social isolation	Blood pressure
Hyperglycemia	Rising pulse
Hypoglycemia	Lack of appetite
	Pacing the room
	T 97.4°F (36.3°C)
	Had insulin injection

Scenario

The following day, the client is relaxed, and the family has arrived at the bedside.

Health History	Nurses' Notes	Healthcare Provider Orders	Vital Signs

Day 3

Vital Signs	0800
Temperature (F/C)	97.4°/36.3°
Heart Rate (bpm)	72
Respirations (bpm)	16
Blood Pressure (mmHg)	118/62

Nurses' Notes

0830: Client's morning blood sugar is 135 mg/dL. Client states is feeling much better this morning and looking forward to going home later today. Client's parents have been told by the NP that client will be going home on insulin injected SubQ and will have a blood glucose monitor. The diabetic educator has been in to provide discharge teaching yesterday, and will come in again today prior to discharge.

1. NGN Item Type: Drop-Down Cloze

30.4.1 The practical nurse reinforces *insulin* teaching to the client and their parents. Choose the *most likely* options for the information missing from the statement that follows by selecting from the list of options provided.

If your blood sugar is _____1_____, have a snack, and if your blood sugar is _____2_____, give insulin as prescribed. At some point, you may want to talk to your PHCP about _____3_____, which is more automated to give hands-free blood glucose control. When you leave today, we'll send you home with _____4_____. It is important that you _____5_____ insulin injection sites. You will have _____6_____ of long-acting insulin to last throughout the day and a _____7_____ of rapid-acting insulin to fine-tune your blood glucose measurement results.

Options for 1, 2, 3	Options for 4, 5, 6, 7
postprandial	correction dose
an insulin pump	metformin
< 70 mg/dL	an insulin pen
Sulfonylureas	rotate
> 200 mg/dL	massage
	a basal dose
	an IV dose
	an oral dose

2. NGN Item Type: Extended Multiple Response Select N

30.4.2 Select the four client statements which indicate *successful* outcomes.
- "I'll be careful when I dial my dose of insulin into the pen injector."
- "I'll need to take extra vitamins and minerals."
- "I can still play sports as long as I work with my PHCP around my insulin needs."
- "The symptoms of hypoglycemia are fruity breath, deep respirations, and increased thirst and hyperglycemic signs are irritability, sweating, tremors, and increased hunger."
- "When I'm at school I'll need to bring an extra mid-afternoon snack."
- "I'll need to dilute my insulin so I don't get too much."
- "My monitor for blood glucose requires only a very little drop of blood."

31

Gastroenteritis

Outcome

The student will use clinical judgment in nursing management of a patient with a gastrointestinal disorder.

Scenario

L.M. is a 9-month-old client brought to the pediatrician's office by L.M.'s father. The father picked up L.M. early from daycare 2 days ago after an episode of vomiting. L.M. is admitted to the local hospital pediatric unit.

Health History	Nurses' Notes	Healthcare Provider Orders	Laboratory Results

L.M. was a 38-week gestation measuring 6 lb, 6 oz, 20 inches long. Client has been solely bottle-fed for the last 3 months since mom returned to work. Client has had diarrhea and vomiting for the last 36 hours. L.M. has had four liquid diaper changes today and last vomited 3 hours ago.

Health History	Nurses' Notes	Healthcare Provider Orders	Laboratory Results

Vital Signs	1650
Temperature (F/C)	100.1°/37.8°
Heart Rate (bpm)	126
Respirations (bpm)	36
Blood Pressure (mmHg)	90/52

Nurses' Notes

1650: Client is sleepy and fussy and opens eyes when dad calls client's name. Dad states there have been fewer diaper changes than normal except for the diarrhea. Assessment: lungs clear to auscultation, skin pale, cool, and smooth, lethargic, hyperactive bowel sounds and decreased skin turgor.

1. NGN Item Type: Multiple Response Grouping

31.1.1 For each body system below, use a checkmark to specify the findings that require immediate follow-up. (Each category must have at least one response option selected.)

Category	Finding
Neurological	• Sleepy
	• Opens his eyes when dad calls his name
	• Lethargic
	• T 100.1°F (37.8°C)
Gastrointestinal	• Hyperactive bowel sounds
	• Diarrhea
	• Vomiting
Integumentary	• Pale
	• Skin cool
	• Skin smooth
	• Decreased skin turgor
	• Diaper rash

2. NGN Item Type: Matrix Multiple Choice

31.1.2 Use an X to indicate which potential issues listed in the left column may place this client at highest risk while in the hospital.

Potential Issue	Risk to Patient
Electrolyte imbalance	
Metabolic acidosis	
Dehydration	
Respiratory distress	
Imbalanced nutrition	
Infection	

Scenario

Several hours later on the evening shift, L.M. is sleeping. The nurse makes rounds and documents in the chart.

Health History	Nurses' Notes	Healthcare Provider Orders	Laboratory Results

Nurses' Notes

1935: IV fluid bolus has been hung by the RN. L.M. is sleeping with mother at bedside. Client's abdomen is nontender, client has not vomited since arrival on unit, and diaper is dry. T is currently 100°F (37.7°C). Client's current weight is 18 lb 12 oz, mom reports weight at 9-month checkup at 20 lb 2 oz.

1. NGN Item Type: Drop-Down Cloze

31.2.1 Choose the *most likely* options for the information missing from the statements below by selecting from the lists of options provided.

Based on the client's current condition, the client's **priority** need will be to prevent _____1_____.

In addition, L.M. will need interventions to prevent _____2_____ and _____2_____ .

Options for 1	Options for 2
Steatorrhea	Failure to thrive
Dehydration	Pneumonia
Constipation	Weight gain
	Fluid and electrolyte imbalance
	Anemia

2. NGN Item Type: Multiple Response Grouping

31.2.2 Select the anticipated HCP orders that the nurse needs to prioritize right away from each of the following categories. (Each category must have at least one response option selected.)

Category	Orders
Medications	• NS IV 34 mL/hr
	• Oxybutynin 5 mg po once a day
	• Acetaminophen suspension (5 mL = 160 mg) 2.5 mL po Q 6 hrs prn fever > T 100.4°F (38°C)
	• Probiotics IV
	• Ceftriaxone 300 mg IV every 12 hours
Nursing interventions	• Decrease sugar and milk intake
	• Daily weight
	• Prepare for surgery
	• Encourage breastfeeding
	• Culture and sensitivity
	• NPO
	• Prepare NG tube for placement

Scenario

Three hours later, both parents are at the bedside where L.M. remains somewhat lethargic. The LVN is caring for L.M. and is explaining the care being provided. The nurse tells the parents the last vomiting has been several hours, and a diaper change with a watery liquid stool has just been completed.

1. NGN Item Type: Multiple Response Select All That Apply

31.3.1 What nursing actions are appropriate for the patient at this time? Select all that apply.
A. Reinforce teaching on handwashing to parents
B. Frequent diaper changes
C. Weigh diapers
D. Apple juice once introducing fluids
E. Vital signs every 2 hours
F. Assess and document vomitus and stools
G. Assess for currant jelly-like stools
H. Provide oral hydration such as Pedialyte as prescribed and tolerated
I. Reintroduce formula slowly once vomiting and diarrhea have ceased

Scenario

The following morning, the nurse documents in the nurses' notes.

Health History	Nurses' Notes	Healthcare Provider Orders	Laboratory Results

Day 2
1030: Client has not vomited in 9 hours and has been able to keep down small amounts of water. Within last 30 minutes has kept down 3 oz of Pedialyte. Nonelastic skin turgor is noted on lower forearm. Child is smiling and interacting with parents. Diaper changed with soft blobs of brown stool with some mushy stool visible. Perianal tissue shows increased erythema. This morning's weight 19 lb 3 oz.

1. NGN Item Type: Highlight Text

31.4.1 Highlight the findings in the nurses' notes the next morning that indicate that L.M. is progressing as expected.

Health History	Nurses' Notes	Healthcare Provider Orders	Laboratory Results

Day 2

1030: Client has not vomited in 9 hours and has been able to keep down small amounts of water. Within last 30 minutes has kept down 3 oz of Pedialyte. Nonelastic skin turgor is noted on lower forearm. Child is smiling and interacting with parents. Diaper changed with soft blobs of brown stool with some mushy stool visible. Perianal tissue shows increased erythema. This morning's weight 19 lb 3 oz.

Pediatric Fracture

32

Scenario

The LVN works at a pediatric hospital in the emergency department. They see an 11-year-old wheel in on a gurney from an ambulance. The mom has not arrived yet, because she had to drop her other children off on her way to the hospital.

Health History	Nurses' Notes	Vital Signs	

11-year-old arrived on gurney via ambulance. Patient is in the trauma bay screaming in pain while holding left upper arm. Report from EMS states the client was riding a bicycle and lost control and ran into a tree. EMS placed gauze dressings over abrasions and noticed the left arm was deformed so they splinted it. Patient's mother told EMS that the patient has no medical history and no known medication allergies.

Health History	Nurses' Notes	Vital Signs	

Patient appears uncomfortable in trauma bay. Vital signs stable on room air. Patient complains their left arm "hurts really bad" and is unable to use a pain scale. Patient also complains of nausea. The left upper arm appears deformed, and radial pulses and pedal pulses are equal bilaterally. There are no other apparent deformities. The left upper arm splint is falling off and saturated with blood. The patient is able to move all fingers and toes, and feels tingling in their left hand.

Health History	Nurses' Notes	Vital Signs	

Heart rate (bpm)	100
Blood pressure (bpm)	98/62
Respiratory rate	22 per minute
SPO$_2$	97% on room air
Temperature	98.0°F (36.7°C)

---

1. NGN Item Type: Hot Spot

32.1.1 Highlight the assessment findings that require follow-up by the nurse.

☐ Patient complains of nausea
☐ Heart rate 100
☐ Blood pressure 98/62
☐ Respiratory rate is 22 per minute and SPO$_2$ is 97% on room air
☐ Temperature is 98.0°F (36.7°C)
☐ Left upper arm deformity
☐ Patient complains left arm "hurts really bad" and unable to use pain scale
☐ Radial pulses and pedal pulses are equal bilaterally
☐ No other apparent deformities
☐ Left upper arm splint is falling off and saturated with blood
☐ Patient is able to move all fingers and toes
☐ Feels tingling in left hand

2. NGN Item Type: Drop-Down Cloze

32.1.2 Choose the *most likely options* for the information missing from the statements below by selecting from the list of options provided.

Based on the assessment findings, the LVN sees the saturated bandage is due to _____1_____, which is of great concern. They also believe the deformed extremity means there is a _____2_____. These findings lead the LVN to understand the injury is most likely a _____3_____.

Options for 1	Options for 2	Options for 3
anticoagulant therapy	congenital defect	closed fracture
the loose dressing	fractured bone	open fracture
hemorrhaging	osteosarcoma	greenstick fracture

Scenario

The LVN is caring for the patient in the postanesthesia care unit (PACU). The pediatric patient has had surgery and is being cared for by the LVN.

Health History	Nurses' Notes	Vital Signs	

An 11-year-old arrived on gurney via ambulance with no medical history and no known medication allergies. X-ray revealed a fracture of the humerus. The patient underwent an open reduction internal fixation (ORIF) for a compound fracture of the humerus. Patient received general anesthesia and the physician applied a cast after the surgery. The plan is to discharge patient home.

Health History	Nurses' Notes	Vital Signs	

1300: Patient's vital signs are stable on room air. Respirations are even and unlabored.

Health History	Nurses' Notes	Vital Signs	

Heart rate (bpm)	109
Blood pressure (bpm)	102/67
Respiratory rate	24 per minute
SPO$_2$	96% on room air
Temperature	98.0°F (36.7°C)

1. NGN Item Type: Drop-Down Cloze

32.2.1 Choose the *most likely option* for the information missing from the statements below by selecting from the list of options provided. Each of the options can only be used once.

The LVN is prioritizing care for the pediatric patient postoperatively. Based on the history of present injury, they see the patient is at a very high risk for a _____1_____ because of the _____2_____. If untreated, the patient could develop _____3_____, so they suspect the physician will order a _____6_____. The LVN recognizes the patient is also a high risk for a _____4_____ because they have a _____5_____ postoperatively.

Options for 1, 2, 3, 4, 5, 6. **Each option can only be used once**
compound fracture
osteomyelitis
cast
compartment syndrome
infection
broad-spectrum antibiotic

2. NGN Item Type: Matrix Multiple Choice

32.2.2 The LVN is planning care for the patient. For each potential nursing intervention, use an X whether the intervention is indicated or contraindicated for care of this pediatric patient with a fracture.

Potential Intervention	Indicated	Contraindicated
Make sure arm remains in the dependent position		
Use distraction techniques		
Administer weight-based dose of pain medication		
Elevate extremity		
Keep patient on bedrest		
Apply ice to surgical site		
Request PCA for patient		
Encourage NSAIDs		
Discuss with parent the child's risk for opiate addiction		
Use FLACC pain scale		

Scenario

The patient's family is at bedside. The MD has written discharge instructions, and the RN educated the patient and family member. The LVN is now at the bedside reinforcing the discharge teaching.

Health History	Nurses' Notes	Vital Signs	

An 11-year-old arrived on gurney via ambulance with no medical history and no known medication allergies. X-ray revealed a fracture of the humerus. The patient underwent an open reduction internal fixation (ORIF) for a compound fracture of the humerus. Patient received general anesthesia and the physician applied a cast after the surgery.

Health History	Nurses' Notes	Vital Signs	

1300: Patient's vital signs are stable on room air. Respirations are even and unlabored.
1400: Patient's mother is at bedside. Patient states pain is 1/10 on numeric scale, so the RN is preparing the patient for discharge.

Health History	Nurses' Notes	Vital Signs	

Heart rate (bpm)	104
Blood pressure (bpm)	100/68
Respiratory rate	22 per minute
SPO$_2$	96% on room air
Temperature	98.0°F (36.7°C)

1. NGN Item Type: Multiple Response Select All That Apply

32.3.1 The LVN discusses which of the following information when they reinforce discharge teaching? Select all that apply.

A. Take pain medication on a regular schedule.
B. Take 81 mg aspirin each day on an empty stomach to prevent DVT.
C. Keep arm elevated as much as possible.
D. Do not move fingers while in cast.
E. Call provider immediately if pain is not controlled by medication, ice, and elevation.
F. Call 9-1-1 if patient experiences chest pain or shortness of breath.
G. Call provider immediately if client loses feeling in fingers.

2. NGN Item Type: Multiple Response Select All That Apply

32.3.2 When the LVN is reinforcing discharge teaching, they realize the patient and family <u>need further instructions</u> when the patient's family states: Select all that apply.

A. "They can go back to playing sports and riding their bike next week."

B. "They need to eat foods high in fiber because of the pain medicine."

C. "They can lift up to 10 pounds with the surgical arm."

D. "I will make sure they do NOT take any aspirin."

E. "They should take the antibiotics only if they get a fever."

F. "They should elevate their extremity as much as possible."

G. "I will make sure they go to the follow-up appointment as scheduled."

H. "They should avoid going to school until the cast is removed."

I. "If I notice a foul smell coming from the cast, I will call the provider."

J. "If their hand or arm turns red and warmer than the other arm, I should call the provider."

33

Meningitis

Outcome

The student will apply critical thinking to planning care for a client with meningitis.

Scenario

A 12-year-old client attending summer camp walks to the camp nurse's office saying, "I feel really bad" with a headache, dizziness, nausea, and feels weak all over. The client's friend says the client is acting "goofy." The camp nurse checks the vital signs: T 101.5°F (38.6°C), P 92, R 18, BP 114/64. The client's mother is notified and takes the client to the local ED. The nurse in the ED settles the client and mother in an exam room, documents, and checks for orders.

Health History	Nurses' Notes	Healthcare Provider Orders	Laboratory Results

1530:
Rash noted on client's extremities. Client states has difficulty moving neck and has some pain in their joints. Current weight: 86 pounds. T 103°F (39.4°C). Client says they thought they had caught a cold earlier in the week.

Health History	Nurses' Notes	Healthcare Provider Orders	Laboratory Results

Lumbar puncture
Blood cultures × 2
Complete blood count

1. NGN Item Type: Drop-Down Cloze

33.1.1 Choose the *most likely* options for the information missing from the statement below by selecting from the list of options provided.

The assessment findings that require **immediate** follow-up include _____1_____, _____2_____, and _____3_____.

Options for 1	Options for 2	Options for 3
BP 114/64	Weight 86 lb	Had a cold
T 103°F (39.4°C)	Nausea	Rash on the extremities
Acting "goofy"	Difficulty moving neck	Headache

2. NGN Item Type: Multiple Response Select All That Apply

33.1.2 Which nursing assessment findings support the client's probable diagnosis of meningitis? Select all that apply.

  A. Headache and nausea
  B. Dizziness
  C. Irritability
  D. P 92 and R 18
  E. BP 114/64
  F. Rash on extremities

G. Difficulty moving neck
H. Pain in joints
I. Weight 86 pounds
J. T 103°F (39.4°C)

Scenario

The client is admitted to the pediatric ICU. Diagnostic tests indicate bacterial meningitis, strongly suggestive of *Neisseria meningitidis*.

1. NGN Item Type: Multiple Choice

33.2.1 Based on the client's current condition, the client's priority need will be to prevent which of the following complications?
A. Seizures
B. Cerebral palsy
C. Autism
D. Infection

2. NGN Item Type: Multiple Response Grouping

33.2.2 Select the anticipated HCP orders from each of the following categories. (Each category must have at least one response option selected.)

Category	Orders
Medications	• Dexamethasone 4 mg IV push just prior to ampicillin
	• Ceftriaxone 1900 mg IV Q 12 hrs
	• Acetaminophen 325 mg po Q 4 hrs prn fever > T 38°C
	• Phenytoin 100 mg po BID
Nursing interventions	• Respiratory isolation precautions
	• 0.9% NS IV at 70 mL/hr
	• Neuro checks every shift
	• Intake and output
	• Stimulating environment
	• Oxygen to keep saturations > 94%
	• Seizure precautions
	• Assist RN with cranial nerve assessment

Scenario

That evening, both parents are at the bedside. The client is sleepy and irritable and states, "I just really wants to go home to see my dog." The client's parents ask questions about the plan of care.

1. NGN Item Type: Multiple Response Select All That Apply

33.3.1 Which of the following are appropriate for the LVN to reinforce with the family at this time? Select all that apply.
A. Keep room lights low
B. Provide a calm and quiet environment
C. Decrease tactile stimulation

   D. Isolation will need to be continued for 7 days
   E. Once client is ready, clear liquids will be started
   F. The client is on contact precaution
   G. Recommend the meningococcal vaccine once recovered

Scenario

The following afternoon, the nurse evaluates the outcomes of the client's treatment plan.

Health History	Nurses' Notes	Healthcare Provider Orders	Laboratory Results

Day 2
1430: T 99.5°F (37.5°C), pain 1/10 on 0 to 10 rating scale, oxygen 2 L/m with O_2 saturation 93%. Client really wants to go home and states dog's name is Buffy. Client denies joint pain and stiffness. Urinary output last 8 hours is 450 mL.

1. NGN Item Type: Matrix Multiple Choice

33.4.1 For each assessment finding, use an X to indicate whether the interventions were <u>effective</u> (helped to meet expected outcomes), <u>ineffective</u> (did not help to meet expected outcomes), or <u>unrelated</u> (not related to the expected outcomes). Each row must have only one option selected.

Assessment Finding	Effective	Ineffective	Unrelated
T 99.5°F (37.5°C) this morning			
Pain 1/10 on 0 to 10 rating scale			
Client states dog's name is Buffy			
Urinary output last 12 hours is 450 mL			
Denies joint pain and stiffness			
Oxygen 2 L/m with O_2 saturation 93%			

Outcome

Organize and interpret patient and family information to provide nursing interventions and evaluate the care of the pediatric patient with asthma.

Scenario

A practical nurse is working in a pediatric clinic and takes a client and their parent to an exam room and documents in the chart.

Health History	**Nurses' Notes**	Vital Signs	Laboratory Results

1000: J.B. is a 5-year-old accompanied by a parent presenting to the pediatric clinic. J.B. has a documented health history of allergic rhinitis and the parent notes recent onset of acute episodes of coughing and wheezing, explaining, "these episodes are occurring more frequently after playing outside and it can take a while for J.B. to catch his breath." The parent notes that J.B. is having trouble sleeping and is tired during the day.

The RN notes: J.B. is sneezing with some congestion but does not appear to be in immediate distress. Child is active in the exam room and is holding a stuffed toy dog.

Health History	Nurses' Notes	**Vital Signs**	Laboratory Results

1000: Vital signs: temperature 98.2°F (36.8°C), pulse 80 beats per minute, respirations 20 breaths per minute, pulse oximetry (SpO$_2$) 96% on room air.

J.B. rates pain as a 0/10 using the FACES pain scale.

---

1. NGN Item Type: Multiple Response Select All That Apply

34.1.1 Which pediatric assessment findings require additional follow-up by the nurse? Select all that apply.

    A. Respiratory rate of 20 and oxygen saturation 96%

    B. Trouble sleeping

    C. Heart rate 80

    D. Acute episodes of coughing and wheezing after playing outside

    E. Active in the exam room

    F. Maternal history of childhood asthma

    G. Stuffed toy dog

    H. Sneezing

    I. Nasal congestion

2. NGN Item Type: Matrix Multiple Choice

34.1.2 Use an X to specify which assessment finding is most likely to be indicated with each of the client's health concerns. Each row must have only one response option selected.

Assessment Finding	Asthma	Allergic Rhinitis
Coughing and wheezing		
Trouble sleeping		
Nasal congestion		
Trouble catching breath		
Sneezing		

Scenario

Health History	Nurses' Notes	Vital Signs	Laboratory Results	Healthcare Provider Orders

1030: Assessment confirms diagnosis of pediatric asthma. Pathophysiology reviewed with family. Emphasized importance of symptom management and identifying triggers. Medication use for exacerbation of symptoms discussed, nurse to provide additional instruction on use of a metered-dose inhaler to client and family.

1. NGN Item Type: Drag-and-Drop Rationale

34.2.1 Choose the *most likely options* for the information missing from the statements below by selecting from the lists of options provided.

Based on a new diagnosis of asthma, the nurse recognizes the client is at highest risk for _____1_____ as evidenced by _____2_____.

Options for 1	Options for 2
Difficulty breathing	Decreased pulse
Eczema	Gastroesophageal reflux
Pulmonary vasodilation	Exercise testing
Increased surfactant	Coughing and wheezing

2. NGN Item Type: Matrix Multiple Choice

34.2.2 The practical nurse is reviewing the generated plan of care for the pediatric client with a new asthma diagnosis. For each nursing action, use an X to indicate if the intervention is indicated or contraindicated for the plan of care.

Nursing Action	Indicated	Contraindicated
Encourage oral fluids		
Introduce incentive spirometry		
Instruct the client on the vagal maneuver		
Review when and whom to call for help during and asthma attack		
Help client identify asthma triggers		
Teach the client how to use a metered-dose inhaler		
Discourage the use of a spacer for inhalers		
Discuss activities that can be tolerated like basketball		

Scenario

Health History	Nurses' Notes	Vital Signs	Laboratory Results

1045: Instruction by demonstration provided to client and family about the use of a metered-dose inhaler with a spacer when the client has trouble breathing. Client and family verbalize understanding of its use, client return demonstrates how to set up and use a metered-dose inhaler.

1. NGN Item Type: Multiple Response Select All That Apply

34.3.1 When providing client teaching on the use of a metered-dose inhaler, the nurse would include which of the following information? Select all that apply.

A. Take a big deep breath in as you quickly inhale the medication.

B. Breathe out a normal breath, and then place your mouth around the mouthpiece as you slowly breathe in.

C. A spacer attachment allows for more time to breathe the medication in.

D. It is important to use this medication whenever you need it.

E. It is important to rinse your mouth after using your metered-dose inhaler.

F. You should keep your metered-dose inhaler where an adult can get it quickly for you.

G. You do not need to shake the metered-dose inhaler before using.

H. Once you inhale the medication, you should hold your breath and count to 10.

2. NGN Item Type: Multiple Response Select N

34.3.2 The client prepares to leave the clinic; the nurse can evaluate the client's learning from which of the following statements. Select the three client statements that indicate successful outcomes.

A. "I need to pay attention to when it feels hard to breathe and let an adult know."

B. "I need to rinse my mouth out after using the metered-dose inhaler."

C. "I need to take the metered-dose inhaler every day at the same time."

D. "Different things may trigger my asthma and stuffed animals might be one of them."

E. "I may not have asthma my whole life."

Leukemia

Outcome

The student will demonstrate comprehensive application of critical thinking in managing the care of the client with leukemia.

Scenario

J.B., a 3-year-old client, has been brought to the pediatrician's office by their mom, who states J.B. has been tired and looks pale. J.B. has not wanted to play outside and seems to not have any energy. The practical nurse documents the following information:

Health History	Nurses' Notes	Healthcare Provider Orders	Laboratory Results

Vital Signs	**1420**
Temperature (F/C)	100.4°/38°
Heart Rate (bpm)	102
Respirations (bpm)	20
Blood Pressure (mmHg)	93/55

Nurses' Notes 1420

Subjective:
- J.B. states has an older sister who is in school today
- Mom reports J.B. is "eating OK"
- J.B. states legs hurt and points to around both knees

Objective:
- Pallor
- Fatigued and listless
- Bruising in lower extremities bilaterally
- Lungs clear to auscultation
- Abdomen soft, normoactive bowel sounds

1. NGN Item Type: Multiple Response Select N

35.1.1 Use an X for the top five findings that would require immediate follow-up.

Client Findings	Top 5 Findings
T 100.4°F (38°C)	
P 102, R 20, BP 93/55	
Pallor	
Mom states J.B. has been tired and looks pale	
Bruising in lower extremities bilaterally	
J.B. states has an older sister who is in school today	
Mom reports J.B. is eating OK	
J.B. states legs hurt and points to around both knees	

2. NGN Item Type: Multiple Response Select All That Apply

35.1.2 Which nursing assessment findings support the client's probable diagnosis of leukemia? Select all that apply.
- A. Low-grade fever
- B. Female
- C. Age
- D. Pallor
- E. Bruises easily
- F. Lethargy
- G. Has sibling

Scenario

The pediatrician tells the mother that they suspect leukemia and admits J.B. to the hospital for further workup. J.B. has had labs drawn and a bone marrow biopsy. The nurse checks the chart for lab results and new orders.

Health History	Nurses' Notes	Healthcare Provider Orders	Laboratory Results

Lab Test	Client	Normal
White blood cell count	WBC 28,260 mm³	4.5 to 11.0 mm³

Health History	Nurses' Notes	Healthcare Provider Orders	Laboratory Results

Diagnosis: Acute lymphocytic leukemia (ALL)
Consult pediatric oncologist

1. NGN Item Type: Drop-Down Cloze

35.2.1 Choose the *most likely* options for the information missing from the statements below by selecting from the lists of options provided.

Based on the client's current treatment plan, the client's **priority** need will be to prevent _____1_____. Other needs that may develop in the near future include _____2_____, _____2_____, and _____2_____.

Options for 1	Options for 2
Alopecia	Anemia
Atelectasis	Pruritis
Infection	Bleeding
	Edema
	Dysrhythmias
	Fractures

2. NGN Item Type: Matrix Multiple Choice

35.2.2 Use an X to indicate which actions listed in the left column would be included in the plan of care to reduce the risk of infection for this client.

Nursing Actions	Implementation
Initiate protective isolation, including wearing masks	
Check mucous membranes and skin puncture sites for signs of infection	
Provide a quiet dark room	
Ensure adequate hydration	
Monitor the client's temperature daily	
Encourage cough and deep breathing	
Check the child's pupillary response	
Teach family members how to carefully wash hands	
Monitor the urine output for color and cloudiness	
Assist the child with frequent oral hygiene and daily bathing	

Scenario

J.B. is started on chemotherapy, with plans for radiation later in their treatment. The client is given 2 units of packed red blood cells by the RN, and their blood counts are improving. The RN and practical nurse collaborate on planning care for J.B.

1. NGN Item Type: Matrix Multiple Choice

35.3.1 Use an X to indicate which actions listed in the left column would be included in the plan of care for this client.

Nursing Actions	Implementation
Monitor VS carefully for changes	
Offer foods high in protein and calories	
Encourage the child to verbalize their feelings	
Use commercial mouthwash often for a dry mouth	
Assist the RN with blood transfusions as needed	
Teach the parents to avoid people who are sick	
Work with the RN to refer the family to a support group	
Assess for lumps above the clavicle	
Teach the parents how to prevent chemotherapy-induced hair loss	

Scenario

The following day, the practical nurse evaluates the client and documents in the nurses' notes.

Health History	Nurses' Notes	Healthcare Provider Orders	Laboratory Results

Day 2

1400: Temperature this afternoon T 100.5°F (38°C). No signs/symptoms of infections noted, with WBC count 12,400 mm^3. Mom and dad are able to teach back the signs and symptoms of infection that need to be reported to the PHCP. J.B. short of breath when sitting up in chair, put back to bed and RN notified. Noted blood on the pillowcase after the afternoon nap. Adequate hydration with urine output WNL. J.B. states abdomen hurts today. Mom states she will make sure J.B. gets into clinic after discharge for their chickenpox vaccination.

1. NGN Item Type: Highlight Text

35.4.1 Highlight the findings in the nurse's notes that would <u>not</u> indicate successful outcomes.

Health History	Nurses' Notes	Healthcare Provider Orders	Laboratory Results

Day 2

1400: Temperature this afternoon T 100.5°F (38°C). No signs/symptoms of infections noted, with WBC count 12,400 mm^3. Mom and dad are able to teach back the signs and symptoms of infection that need to be reported to the PHCP. J.B. short of breath when sitting up in chair, put back to bed and RN notified. Noted blood on the pillowcase after the afternoon nap. Adequate hydration with urine output WNL. J.B. states abdomen hurts today. Mom states she will make sure J.B. gets into clinic after discharge for their chickenpox vaccination.

Anxiety

Outcome

The student will be able to integrate clinical judgment in planning, implementing, and evaluating care of the client with anxiety.

Scenario

A 40-year-old client is in the clinic to see their primary healthcare provider (PHCP). The practical nurse gathers initial data prior to the PCHP coming into the room.

Health History	Nurses' Notes	Healthcare Provider Orders	Vital Signs

Vital Signs	1030
Temperature (F/C)	97.8°/36.5°
Heart Rate (bpm)	98
Respirations (bpm)	20
Blood Pressure (mmHg)	160/88
Height	5'5"
Weight	146
BMI	24.3

Health History	Nurses' Notes	Healthcare Provider Orders	Vital Signs

1030: Client states is going through a divorce and worries about everything all the time. The client has two daughters ages 10 and 12. Client decided to come in because they told their daughter last week she couldn't go to her best friend's house for a birthday party sleep-over next month because something bad could happen. "What if she gets kidnapped or gets lost?" The client's mother lives a couple of miles away and is at their house often. The client works as a receptionist at a busy office. Client reports their mind is "like a hamster on a hamster wheel." Client states can't get thoughts out of their mind and is constantly exhausted. The client is visibly trembling and foot bounces while talking.

1. NGN Item Type: Highlight Text

36.1.1 Highlight the assessment findings that require follow-up by the nurse.

Health History	Nurses' Notes	Healthcare Provider Orders	Vital Signs

Vital Signs	1030
Temperature (F/C)	97.8°/36.5°
Heart Rate (bpm)	98
Respirations (bpm)	20
Blood Pressure (mmHg)	160/88
Height	5'5"
Weight	146
BMI	24.3

Health History	Nurses' Notes	Healthcare Provider Orders	Vital Signs

1030: Client states is going through a divorce and worries about everything all the time. The client has two daughters ages 10 and 12. Client decided to come in because they told their daughter last week she couldn't go to her best friend's house for a birthday party sleep-over next month because something bad could happen. "What if she gets kidnapped or gets lost?" The client's mother lives a couple of miles away and is at their house often. The client works as a receptionist at a busy office. Client reports their mind is "like a hamster on a hamster wheel." Client states can't get thoughts out of their mind and is constantly exhausted. The client is visibly trembling and foot bounces while talking.

2. NGN Item Type: Multiple Response Select All That Apply

36.1.2 The LPN will ask which priority questions to gather additional information about the client's highest priority needs? Select all that apply

- A. "Do you have periods of extreme sadness?"
- B. "Do you get headaches or muscle tension?"
- C. "Why would you want your daughter to miss her friend's party?"
- D. "Have you ever thought about harming yourself?"
- E. "Do you have trouble concentrating at work or at home?"
- F. "Are you having trouble falling asleep or staying asleep?"

Scenario

After seeing the NP, the client refuses treatment but agrees to return to the clinic in a few weeks. Four weeks later when she returns, the LPN documents the following information.

Health History	Nurses' Notes	Healthcare Provider Orders	Vital Signs

Vital Signs	1300
Temperature (F/C)	98.4°/36.8°
Heart Rate (bpm)	110
Respirations (bpm)	24
Blood Pressure (mmHg)	180/102

Health History	Nurses' Notes	Healthcare Provider Orders	Vital Signs

1300: Client paces the room and states had to wait almost 30 minutes in the waiting room and is sure the NP has found something wrong. Client states has felt heart is racing and sometimes has to curl up on the floor next to the bed because they are so scared. The client reports waking up at night with a hot flush and in a cold sweat and can't think straight. Client states this is happening more and more and now is worried they can't pay their bills and that their kids will be taken away.

1. NGN Item Type: Drop-Down Cloze

36.2.1 Choose the *most likely options* for the information missing from the statements below by selecting from the lists of options provided.

The client is most likely experiencing a ___1___. The priority at this time will be to promote ___2___ and ___3___.

Options for 1	Options for 2	Options for 3
Phobia	Decreased subjective distress	Self-esteem
Panic attack/disorder	Acceptance	Insomnia
Obsessive-compulsive disorder	Fatigue	Return of VS to baseline

Scenario

The LPN speaks to the client in a low-pitched voice with a calm manner. The NP enters the room and quietly speaks to the client. The client's anxiety is noticeably reduced, and the NP suggests a treatment plan, including medications. After the NP leaves the room, the client begins to ask questions.

1. NGN Item Type: Matrix Multiple Choice

36.3.1 Use an X to indicate which actions listed in the left column that the LPN anticipates will be included in the plan of care for this patient.

Nursing Actions	Implementation
Reinforce teaching of prescribed medications	
Discuss alternative therapies such as meditation, animal therapy, or controlled breathing	
Reinforce problem-solving techniques	
Encourage a glass of wine at night to relax and promote sleep	
Assist the client to understand that anxiety like this may be present for the rest of their life	
Use active listening techniques	
Reinforce exercise such as walking or yoga as a positive coping mechanism	
Encourage the client to find reasons for living	
While the client is in a panic attack, remain with the client and attend to their physical symptoms	

Scenario

The client returns for an appointment with the NP 6 weeks later. The LPN reinforces teaching with the client.

Health History	Nurses' Notes	Healthcare Provider Orders	Vital Signs

Vital Signs	1445
Temperature (F/C)	98.4°/36.8°
Heart Rate (bpm)	86
Respirations (bpm)	16
Blood Pressure (mmHg)	136/72

Health History	Nurses' Notes	Healthcare Provider Orders	Vital Signs

1445: Client states has been taking lorazepam 0.5 mg po tid and sertraline 50 mg po daily. Client reports has seen a therapist and started cognitive behavioral therapy. Client states is starting to feel better so will stop taking the medications.

1. NGN Item Type: Matrix Multiple Choice

36.4.1 Use an X for nursing actions listed below that are <u>indicated</u> (necessary) or <u>contraindicated</u> (could be harmful) for this client. Only one selection can be made for each nursing action.

Nursing Action	Indicated	Contraindicated
"Sertraline can cause GI upset such as nausea, vomiting, diarrhea, or constipation."		
"Lorazepam can make you drowsy so be careful about driving."		
"Always take sertraline on an empty stomach."		
"Monitor your weight once a week."		
"You should be feeling much better within just a week or so."		
"Keep all your appointments with your PHCP."		
"If you miss a dose of your medication, it's OK to take it with your next dose."		
"Continue to decrease your lorazepam dose as the NP prescribed it."		
"Continue to take the sertraline even when you are feeling better."		

Scenario

A month later, the client returns for a follow-up visit. The LPN documents the following information.

Health History	**Nurses' Notes**	Healthcare Provider Orders	Vital Signs

0830: Client reports is sleeping now 7 hours at night. Client states, "I allowed my daughter to go to the sleep-over!" Client reports, "I'm feeling more productive at work and drinking a lot of coffee and cola to help with coping." Client states is taking half the amount of lorazepam and will continue to gradually decrease the dose. Client reports that sometimes is having some pretty upsetting and severe nightmares about the future and still can just feel so hopeless. Reports has been in cognitive behavioral therapy now for several weeks and has learned some great coping strategies and has started doing yoga every evening before bed.

1. NGN Item Type: Matrix Multiple Choice

36.5.1 Use an X to indicate the assessment findings that indicate successful outcomes.

Client Statement	Successful Outcomes
"I am sleeping now 7 hours at night."	
"I allowed my daughter to go to the sleep-over!"	
"I'm feeling more productive at work."	
"I've been drinking a lot of coffee and cola to help me cope."	
"I'm taking half the amount of lorazepam and I'll continue to gradually decrease the dose."	
"Sometimes I have some pretty upsetting and severe nightmares about my future."	
"I've been in cognitive behavioral therapy now for several weeks and I've learned some great coping strategies."	
"I still can just feel so hopeless."	
"I've started doing yoga every evening before bed."	

Bipolar

Outcome

The student will apply principles of the nursing process and clinical judgment in the care of the client with bipolar disease.

Scenario

A 28-year-old client is brought to the ED by the police. They were picked up for driving too fast and going through several red lights. When the police stopped the client, they were very upbeat and talked very loudly and rapidly without pauses. The police recognized a potential mental health issue and brought them to the community hospital. The LVN settles them in the ED room and begins to gather information.

Health History	Nurses' Notes	Healthcare Provider Orders	Vital Signs

2030: The client expresses has not slept in 2 days; "I don't need sleep, I'm not tired and I've never felt better in my life." Client states has been a dental hygienist until a few days ago when they decided they needed to be a writer. Speech is at times unclear, jumbled, with nonsense words and scrambled sentences. The client is restless and moves their hands wildly while they talk. They pull a thick, untidy notebook with scraps of paper falling out of it out of their bag and begin to write feverishly.

1. NGN Item Type: Matrix Multiple Choice

37.1.1 Use an X for the top three findings that would require immediate follow-up.

Patient Findings	Top 3 Findings
Hasn't slept the last 2 nights	
Speech rapid, unclear, and jumbled	
Ran red light	
Restless and moves hands wildly	
Wants to be a writer	
Driving too fast	

2. NGN Item Type: Matrix Multiple Choice

37.1.2 Use an X to indicate which potential issues listed in the left column may place this client at risk while in the hospital.

Potential Issue	Risk to Patient
Delirium	
Dissociative identity disorder	
Risky decision-making	
Delusional thinking	
Hypochondriasis	

Scenario

The client has been seen by the psychiatric NP in the emergency department and orders have been written. While waiting for transfer, the client laughs frequently and tells the LVN that they are writing a really important movie script and have been awake for the last 3 days to write. When the LVN asks if they could read a little of it, the client is delighted to share it. In the notebook, the LVN finds words and thoughts are scribbled in a variety of directions and are nonsensical. The client is transferred to the unit.

Health History	Nurses' Notes	Healthcare Provider Orders	Vital Signs

2145:
- Admit to mental health unit
- Diagnosis: bipolar
- Divalproex sodium 250 mg po bid
- Trazadone 50 mg po Q HS

1. NGN Item Type: Drop-Down Cloze

37.2.1 Choose the *most likely* options for the information missing from the statements below by selecting from the lists of options provided.

Based on the patient's current treatment plan, the patient's **priority** need will be to prevent _____1_____. Other priorities of care include _____2_____, _____2_____, and _____2_____.

Options for 1	Options for 2
Electroconvulsive therapy	Mood stabilization
Hygiene deficits	Reinforcing nonritualistic behaviors
Suicide	Achieve the highest level of functioning
	Ensure compliance with medications
	Speaking softly or whispering
	Identify splitting behavior

2. NGN Item Type: Multiple Response Select N

37.2.2 Which of the following *five* nursing interventions would the LVN anticipate will be included in the plan of care?
- ☐ Spend time with client discussing the client's worth and value
- ☐ Give instructions clearly and repeat as necessary
- ☐ Establish a schedule with client for sleeping
- ☐ Collaborate with the RN to develop a no harm contract
- ☐ Administer oral medications as ordered
- ☐ Use active listening
- ☐ Set limits on compulsive behaviors that may interfere with well-being

Scenario

Three days later, the client's mood appears to be stabilizing. They have slept for several hours each night and their speech is slower and more coherent. The client continues to write their script.

1. NGN Item Type: Matrix Multiple Choice

37.3.1 Use an X to indicate which actions listed in the left column would be included in the plan of care for this patient.

Nursing Actions	Implementation
Keep client away from others for safety.	
Reinforce teaching to client on taking medications on schedule.	
Remind client divalproex sodium is a mood stabilizer and needs consistent blood levels.	
Collaborate with the RN case manager for an outpatient provider schedule.	
Remind client to avoid triggers that can contribute to mania.	
Reinforce teaching on safety such as not driving during manic episode.	
Administer tranquilizer medications to assist in controlling behavior.	
Divalproex sodium can cause transient nausea and drowsiness.	

Scenario

Seven days later, the LVN documents the client's progression.

Health History	Nurses' Notes	Healthcare Provider Orders	Vital Signs

Day 8 1130: Client's mood appears to have stabilized. Slept 6 hours during the night. Energy has waned, pressured speech is absent. Client states is no longer writing the movie script. This morning client talked with boss at work and has discussed returning to work once completely stabilized.

1. NGN Item Type: Multiple Response Select All That Apply

37.4.1 Which of the following findings indicate successful outcomes? Select all that apply.
A. Client has abided by the no harm contract.
B. Client states it will be fine to occasionally stay up all night.
C. Client has agreed to continue on their medications and has set up reminders in their phone.
D. This morning's divalproex sodium level is within therapeutic range.
E. Client is pacing and talking loudly.
F. Client states the need to pay close attention to their sleep patterns.
G. Client has decided not to share information about their disorder with their family and friends.
H. Client states importance of staying on schedule with mental health provider office visits.
I. Client states that now they're on their medications, having caffeine and alcohol won't make any difference.

Outcome

The student will prioritize the key aspects of nursing management of the client with depression.

Scenario

A 56-year-old client comes to the healthcare providers (HCP) clinic for a check-up. The practical nurse settles the client in an exam room and documents findings in the computer.

Health History	Nurses' Notes	Healthcare Provider Orders	Vital Signs

Client is 56 years old with a history of hysterectomy and depression. Client states has been depressed on and off since age 21. The client is a high school graduate who has worked as a clerk in the same office for over 15 years. Client lives alone in a townhouse. Denies drug use and reports occasional alcohol intake.

Health History	Nurses' Notes	Healthcare Provider Orders	Vital Signs

1600: Client states was feeling better and stopped taking medications, client states has done that multiple times over the years. Client has decreased eye contact, is tearful, and appears tired. Client reports a lack of interest in anything and can't be bothered to eat, reporting a recent 5- or 6-lb weight loss. Client states, "I'll never be happy." Reports is in bed a lot but doesn't ever feel has slept well. States has worked in the same place "forever," states does not have any friends there now. Lungs are clear, heart rate and rhythm are regular, abdomen soft and nontender. Client had recent lab work drawn, which shows sodium, potassium, glucose, creatinine, and TSH all within normal limits.

1. NGN Item Type: Highlight Text

38.1.1 Highlight the assessment findings above that require follow-up by the nurse.

Health History	Nurses' Notes	Healthcare Provider Orders	Vital Signs

Client is 56 years old with a history of hysterectomy and depression. Client states has been depressed on and off since age 21. The client is a high school graduate who has worked as a clerk in the same office for over 15 years. Client lives alone in a townhouse. Denies drug use and reports occasional alcohol intake.

Health History	Nurses' Notes	Healthcare Provider Orders	Vital Signs

1600: Client states was feeling better and stopped taking medications, client states has done that multiple times over the years. Client has decreased eye contact, is tearful, and appears tired. Client reports a lack of interest in anything and can't be bothered to eat, reporting a recent 5- or 6-lb weight loss. Client states, "I'll never be happy." Reports is in bed a lot but doesn't ever feel has slept well. States has worked in the same place "forever," states does not have any friends there now. Lungs are clear, heart rate and rhythm are regular, abdomen soft and nontender. Client had recent lab work drawn, which shows sodium, potassium, glucose, creatinine, and TSH all within normal limits.

2. NGN Item Type: Matrix Multiple Choice

38.1.2 Use an X to indicate which potential issues listed in the left column may place this client at risk.

Potential Issue	Risk to Patient
Problems with coping	
Nausea	
Personal injury	
Hopelessness	
Anxiety	
Infection	
Loneliness	

Scenario

The client continues to be tearful throughout the appointment. The client states that they are so lonely and feels hopeless and worthless. The client reports that they have called in sick to work three times in the last 2 weeks, and they don't think anyone even noticed they were gone. The client tearfully states that there really is nothing much to live for.

Health History	Nurses' Notes	Healthcare Provider Orders	Vital Signs

Duloxetine 60 mg po daily
Referral for cognitive behavioral therapy (CBT)

1. NGN Item Type: Drop-Down Cloze

38.2.1 Choose the *most likely* options for the information missing from the statements below by selecting from the lists of options provided.

The client is at the **highest** risk for developing _____1_____ as evidenced by the client's _____2_____, _____2_____, _____2_____, and _____2_____.

Options for 1	Options for 2
Ineffective coping	Living alone
Social isolation	Feelings of worthlessness
Suicidal thoughts	Lack of interest
	Decreased eye contact
	Nothing to live for
	Weight loss
	Occasional alcohol intake
	Lack of social support
	History of depression

2. NGN Item Type: Matrix Multiple Choice

38.2.2 Use an X for the nursing actions listed below that are <u>indicated</u> (appropriate or necessary) or <u>contraindicated</u> (could be harmful) for the client's care at this time. Only one selection can be made for each nursing action.

Nursing Action	Indicated	Contraindicated
Reinforce need to check blood pressure or have it checked frequently		
Remind client they will be able to stop their medication after 4 to 9 months		
Encourage the client to attend CBT to correct self-thoughts		
Provide nonjudgmental support		
Reinforce teaching to increase fluids and take medication with food		
Reinforce teaching regarding electroconvulsive therapy (ECT)		
Remind client they'll need to come in to have blood drawn for serum drug levels		
Assess for suicidal thoughts and plan		

Scenario

The client returns to the clinic 8 weeks later for a follow-up visit. The client is relaxed and appears well rested. The practical nurse notices the client maintains eye contact during their conversation with the nurse. The client states they think they are doing everything they need to be doing to feel better.

1. NGN Item Type: Drop-Down Rationale

38.3.1 Choose the *most likely* options for the information missing from the statement below by selecting from the list of options provided.

The practical nursing student would first _____1_____ and then can _____2_____.

Options for 1	Options for 2
Remind the client about the importance of their medication	Plan for an inpatient stay for the client
Perform a full head to toe and mental health assessment	Reinforce teaching as needed
Check the clients' current understanding of treatment plan	Demonstrate relaxing breathing exercises

2. NGN Item Type: Multiple Response Select N

38.3.2 Which of the following *four findings* indicate successful outcomes?
- ☐ Client joined a depression support group.
- ☐ Client states is not sleeping well.
- ☐ Client's weight is up 5 pounds.
- ☐ Client states will stay on the medication through the winter.
- ☐ Client reports "is pretty darned constipated now."
- ☐ Client is looking forward to attending a nephew's wedding.
- ☐ Client's sister has moved closer, and they lunch together every week.

Scenario

The client has spent most of the time sleeping. Two days later, the nurse makes morning rounds and documents assessment findings. The practical nurse collaborates with the RN to make a plan of care.

| Health History | Nurses' Notes | Healthcare Provider Orders | Laboratory Results |

Day 3
0830: Client appears to be declining and is showing increasing alcohol withdrawal symptoms. Client reports experiencing delirium, shakiness, and nausea. Client is tachycardic, fidgety, and diaphoretic. Client states is feeling anxious and does not calm down easily.

1. NGN Item Type: Matrix Multiple Choice

39.3.1 Use an X to indicate which actions listed in the left column would be included in the plan of care for this patient.

Nursing Actions	Implementation
Monitor vital signs every 1 to 4 hours based on the assessment of the sedation/agitation level	
Administer naloxone	
Administer lorazepam 2 mg po Q 4 hrs	
Search client's personal belongings	
Encourage counseling and group support once through the withdrawal symptoms	
Collaborate with the RN for one-on-one sitter at the bedside	
Work with RN to give lorazepam 1 to 2 mg IV Q 4 hrs prn per the assessment of the sedation/agitation level	
Provide empathetic and nonjudgmental communication	

Scenario

Two days later, the client has stabilized and will be discharged home. The client will go home with their parents for the immediate future.

1. NGN Item Type: Matrix Multiple Choice

39.4.1 Prior to discharge, the nurse assesses the following information. Use an X next to the patient statements that indicate successful outcomes.

Patient Statement	Successful Outcomes
"I understand this is not just normal drinking for my age."	
"I will take disulfiram as discussed with my provider."	
"I will drink a lot of extra water every day."	
"I don't think I can do this; I'm really scared."	
"I know I need help and I'll be reaching out to my counselor and involving family and friends in family therapy."	
"I haven't had any shakes or tremors for a couple of days now."	
"I know that if I get sick, I can take cough medicine, it doesn't have a lot of alcohol in it."	

Outcome

The student will demonstrate comprehensive application of critical thinking in managing the care of the client with a sensory disorder.

Scenario

A 78-year-old client has recently moved to a long-term care center assisted living facility after living independently at home. The LPN makes a daily check-in visit and documents the findings.

Health History	Nurses' Notes	Healthcare Provider Orders	Laboratory Results

Client is 78-year-old who recently had a mild CVA with residual mild weakness in left hand. Has been admitted to a long-term care center assisted living facility. Client's spouse is recently deceased. Client has a history of right femur fracture in their late 40s.

Health History	Nurses' Notes	Healthcare Provider Orders	Laboratory Results

1030: Client admits seems to be tripping over things a lot recently and fell last evening over a couch corner. Client states has a daughter and her family who live in a town nearby, but client feels sad and is lonely in this new home. Client states everyone around "can't speak well, they all mumble so that I can't understand their words" and so hasn't gotten involved in anything. Client appears to be having a difficult time understanding what is being said. Client's right hand grip is 5/5, left hand grip is 4/5, right and left foot push/pulls are equal bilaterally at 5/5, and gait is steady and even.

1. NGN Item Type: Matrix Multiple Choice

40.1.1 Use an X to indicate which patient assessment findings require follow-up by the nurse at this time.

Assessment Finding	Assessment Finding That Requires Follow-Up
Tripping over things	
Fell last evening	
Foot push/pulls are equal bilaterally at 5/5	
Gait steady and even	
Sad and is lonely	
People can't speak well and mumble	
Hasn't gotten involved	
Difficult time understanding what is being said	
Right hand grip 5/5	
Left hand grip 4/5	

2. NGN Item Type: Multiple Response Select All That Apply

40.1.2 The LPN will ask which priority questions to gather additional information about the patient's highest priority needs? Select all that apply.

  A. Do you have any history of hearing loss in your family?
  B. Have you noticed any change in your vision?
  C. Do you have any blurred vision or changes in seeing colors?
  D. Do you feel your hearing has decreased?
  E. Why didn't you see the corner of the couch?
  F. Do you have any pain or discomfort in your eyes?
  G. Have you told your daughter about the bruising?
  H. How often do you have to ask people to repeat what they said to you?

Scenario

The LPN notified the RN and NP of their findings with the client. The NP assesses the client and is concerned with both hearing and vision. The client is sent to an audiologist for their hearing, is found to have presbycusis, and has hearing aids ordered. The ophthalmologist discovered cataracts and the client is taken for outpatient cataract surgery on their left eye. The LPN documents in the client's chart.

Health History	Nurses' Notes	Healthcare Provider Orders	Vital Signs

1135: The client is returned to their room following the outpatient eye surgery, daughter is with the client.

1. NGN Item Type: Multiple Response Select N

40.2.1 Based on the patient's current treatment plan, the patient's priority needs will be to prevent which four of the following?

☐ Infection
☐ Ringing or continuous noise in the ear
☐ Increased intraocular pressure
☐ Social withdrawal
☐ "Tunnel" vision
☐ Depression

2. NGN Item Type: Matrix Multiple Choice

40.2.2 Use an X to indicate which actions listed in the left column would be included in the plan of care for this patient.

Nursing Actions	Relevant Nursing Actions
Assist with ambulation after cataract surgery until client has stabilized	
Face the client when speaking	
Remind client to stay in bed and remain as still as possible	
Speak slowly and clearly	
Speak in a higher volume and pitch	
Provide eye patch as ordered postoperatively	
A cochlear implant may be an option to assist with hearing	
Instill eye drops as prescribed	
Assist with safety measures and prevention including for falls	

Scenario

The next morning, the LPN visits the client and the daughter who has stayed the night.

Health History	Nurses' Notes	Healthcare Provider Orders	Vital Signs

1000: The client states is feeling pretty good and is looking forward to the eye patch coming off and to begin using the new hearing aids. Reinforced teaching to the client and daughter.

1. NGN Item Type: Drop-Down Cloze

40.3.1 Choose the *most likely* options for the information missing from the statement below by selecting from the list of options provided.

After cataract surgery, it is important to avoid rubbing the postoperative left eye. An itchy eye and a _____1_____are normal for a few days. Eye drops will be needed several times a day for _____2_____and the staff is happy to assist the client as needed. Presbycusis is a sensorineural hearing loss associated with _____3_____. It will be important to begin using your new hearing aids slowly to adjust to them. As you get used to the hearing aids, we will assist you to adjust the _____4_____ to the minimal hearing level; otherwise, you can get feedback squeaking. It is important to give the hearing aids 2 to 4 full weeks of wearing them daily to see how they can help you and adjustments can be made.

Options for 1,2	Options for 3,4
severe eye pain	on and off switch
2 to 4 weeks	batteries
decreased vision	head injury
6 months	volume
a week	otitis media
little discomfort	hypothyroidism
yellow discharge	aging

Scenario

Two weeks later, the LPN makes their morning rounds and visits the client to assess and evaluate the effectiveness of the treatment plan.

1. NGN Item Type: Matrix Multiple Choice

40.4.1 For each assessment finding, use an X to indicate whether the nursing interventions were <u>effective</u> (helped to meet expected outcomes), <u>ineffective</u> (did not help to meet expected outcomes), or <u>unrelated</u> (not related to the expected outcomes). Only one selection can be made for each nursing action.

Assessment Finding	Effective	Ineffective	Unrelated
Client states they don't wear their hearing aids when family is visiting			
Vision in left eye is improved			
Client has not tripped or fallen			
Client reports left hand grip hasn't improved any			
Has a headache in the front around the sinus area			
Client is not asking "what did you say?"			
Client states played bingo last night			
Client reports they are getting eye drops in at least once a day			

Polypharmacy

Outcome

The student will use clinical judgment in nursing management of the use of multiple medications in an elderly client.

Scenario

An 82-year-old client was brought to the emergency department by their daughter, who reports her parent has been throwing up for several days with new-onset confusion. The practical nurse takes client and daughter to an exam room and documents in the chart.

Health History	Nurses' Notes	Healthcare Provider Orders	Laboratory Results

82-year-old client recently saw primary healthcare provider (PHCP) with a cough, was diagnosed with mild pneumonia.

Client history of diabetes mellitus type 2, heart failure, coronary artery disease, hypertension, and osteoarthritis.

Daughter states parent has a PHCP, a cardiologist, and an orthopedic doctor.

Daughter provides a partial list of medications including furosemide, potassium chloride, metoprolol, aspirin, metformin, and ibuprofen, but there are more at home.

Health History	Nurses' Notes	Healthcare Provider Orders	Laboratory Results

Vital Signs	1345
Temperature (F/C)	97.8°/36.5°
Heart Rate (bpm)	62
Respirations (bpm)	14
Blood Pressure (mmHg)	112/62

Nurses' Notes

1345: Client states has not been eating well lately, doesn't feel like eating. Daughter is sure client has experienced weight loss, and states client has been throwing up and appears to have new-onset confusion. Client verbalizes has tried to keep up with all the medications for years, "but the doctors just keep adding more." Client states has an itchy nose and has been sneezing. The client is unable to tell the practical nurse what the medications are or how they are taken. Client states that they take some at all different times of the day.

Health History	Nurses' Notes	Healthcare Provider Orders	Laboratory Results

Lab Test	Client	Normal
White blood cell count	WBC 8,520 mm^3	4.5–11.0 mm^3
AST	**82** U/L	1–35 U/L
ALT	**74** U/L	4–36 U/L
Hemoglobin	14.2 g/dL	14.0–18.0 g/dL
Hematocrit	42.7%	37.0–54.0 mL/dL

1. NGN Item Type: Highlight Text

41.1.1 Highlight the assessment findings that require follow-up by the nurse.

| Health History | Nurses' Notes | Healthcare Provider Orders | Laboratory Results |

82-year-old client recently saw primary healthcare provider (PHCP) with a cough, was diagnosed with mild pneumonia.

Client history of diabetes mellitus type 2, heart failure, coronary artery disease, hypertension, and osteoarthritis.

Daughter states parent has a PHCP, a cardiologist, and an orthopedic doctor.

Daughter provides a partial list of medications including furosemide, potassium chloride, metoprolol, aspirin, metformin, and ibuprofen, but there are more at home.

| Health History | Nurses' Notes | Healthcare Provider Orders | Laboratory Results |

Vital Signs	1345
Temperature (F/C)	97.8°/36.5°
Heart Rate (bpm)	62
Respirations (bpm)	14
Blood Pressure (mmHg)	112/62

Nurses' Notes

1345: Client states has not been eating well lately, doesn't feel like eating. Daughter is sure client has experienced weight loss and states client has been throwing up and appears to have new-onset confusion. Client verbalizes has tried to keep up with all the medications for years, "but the doctors just keep adding more." Client states has an itchy nose and has been sneezing. The client is unable to tell the practical nurse what the medications are or how they are taken. Client states that they take some at all different times of the day.

| Health History | Nurses' Notes | Healthcare Provider Orders | Laboratory Results |

Lab Test	Client	Normal
White blood cell count	WBC 8,520 mm^3	4.5–11.0 mm^3
AST	**82** U/L	1–35 U/L
ALT	**74** U/L	4–36 U/L
Hemoglobin	14.2 g/dL	14.0–18.0 g/dL
Hematocrit	42.7%	37.0–54.0 mL/dL

2. NGN Item Type: Drop-Down Table

41.1.2 Some of the medications on the list the client's daughter brought in have complete information, and other medications have information missing. Choose the *most likely* options for the information missing from the table below by selecting from the lists of options provided.

Medication	Dose, Route, Frequency	Drug Class	Indication
Furosemide	20 mg oral daily	1	Remove excess fluid
Potassium chloride	2	Mineral/electrolyte	Treat low potassium
Metoprolol	25 mg oral twice daily	Beta-blocker	3
Aspirin	325 mg oral daily	4	Antiplatelet
5	500 mg oral twice daily	Biguanide	Diabetes mellitus type 2
Ibuprofen	6	NSAID	Arthritis pain

Options for 1	Options for 2	Options for 3
Aldosterone antagonist	40 mEq IV daily	Hypertension
Vasodilator	60 mEq oral four times a day	Diabetes
Diuretic	40 mEq oral daily	Osteoarthritis
Options for 4	**Options for 5**	**Options for 6**
Corticosteroid	Insulin	325 mg orally once daily
DMARD	Metformin	200 mg 2 tabs orally four times a day prn pain
NSAID	Glipizide	600 mg orally every 6 hours prn pain

Scenario

The client is admitted to the medical unit. The client's daughter is asked to bring a complete list of all medications. She returns from the client's home with a paper bag of medication bottles. The practical nurse goes over the medications with the client and documents in the nurses' notes the additional list of the client's medications.

Health History	Nurses' Notes	Healthcare Provider Orders	Laboratory Results

1500: Noted one mail-in pharmacy and two local pharmacies listed on the medications.

Additional medications in the bag include:

- Lisinopril 20 mg po daily
- Levofloxacin 500 mg po daily
- Hydrocodone/acetaminophen 5/325 mg po q 4 hrs prn pain

Additional over-the-counter (OTC) medications include:

- Multivitamin ("I take one most mornings")
- Acetaminophen 650 mg ("I take 1 every 4 hours or so as I need it for my arthritis pain")
- Tums ("a few here and there since my stomach has been bothering me")
- Benadryl ("for allergies this time of year")

1. NGN Item Type: Multiple Response Select N

41.2.1 Based on the client's current condition, use an X to indicate which *three* of the client's potential problems listed in the left column that are the *highest priority* to prevent?

Potential Problem	Priority for Prevention
Falls	
Confusion	
Dry mouth	
Toxicity	
Addiction	

2. NGN Item Type: Matrix Multiple Choice

41.2.2 Use an X to indicate which actions listed in the left column would be included in the plan of care for this patient.

Nursing Actions	Relevant Nursing Actions
Reinforce to client they can now take all of their medications at one time	
Reinforce how to take orthostatic BP & pulse as ordered	
Discuss use of weekly or daily medication cassette or pill box	
Encourage client to take their medications with sips of water	
Assist the client to develop a schedule to take their medications	
Encourage the client to use one pharmacy	
Reinforce to client they need to swallow the potassium chloride whole	
Remind the client that they can take all the OTC medications as often as needed since they aren't prescribed	
Encourage the daughter and client to make up a simple chart or list of daily medication schedule	

Scenario

The NP has changed their medications and 3 days later the client has shown steady improvement. The nurse documents in the nurses' notes and checks the chart.

Health History	Nurses' Notes	Healthcare Provider Orders	Laboratory Results

Vital Signs	**1030**
Temperature (F/C)	97.8°/36.5°
Heart Rate (bpm)	74
Respirations (bpm)	16
Blood Pressure (mmHg)	118/68

Nurses' Notes

1030: Client states, "I guess I got a little mixed up." Client's daughter reports that client will need someone to help with medications at home.

Health History	Nurses' Notes	Healthcare Provider Orders	Laboratory Results

Home medications:
- Stop the lisinopril
- Aspirin 81 mg orally daily
- Metoprolol 25 mg orally daily
- Hydrocodone/acetaminophen 5/325 mg orally one every 6 hours as needed for pain
- Furosemide 10 mg orally daily
- Potassium chloride 20 mg orally daily
- Acetaminophen 500 mg orally every 6 hours as needed for pain
- Finish the entire course of levofloxacin, then stop taking
- Stop the ibuprofen
- Stop the Benadryl (recommend second-generation loratadine as needed instead)

Anticipate discharge tomorrow with home health

1. NGN Item Type: Drop-Down Rationale

41.3.1 Choose the *most likely* options for the information missing from the statement below by selecting from the list of options provided.

The practical nurse would first _____1_____ to _____2_____.

Options for 1	Options for 2
Reinforce teaching again regarding all medications	Plan for medication safety at home
Administer pain medications	Make sure client can repeat back all information correctly
Collaborate with the RN for home health referral	To keep pain level at 0/10

2. NGN Item Type: Multiple Response Select N

41.3.2 Which of the following *four findings* indicate successful outcomes?

- ☐ Client to be moved to a long-term care facility to live.
- ☐ The client states they understand why they were hospitalized.
- ☐ The client reports they cannot remember when they should take which medications·at what times.
- ☐ A home health LPN is scheduled to begin home visits tomorrow.
- ☐ The client verbalizes when to call their PHCP for side effects or changes.
- ☐ The daughter and the client made up a list to refer to for answers if the client forgets.
- ☐ The client states they will use their primary pharmacy plus a mail-in pharmacy for just a few medications.

Outcomes

The student will apply principles of the nursing process and clinical judgment in the care of the client with Alzheimer's disease.

Scenario

The client is 74-year-old who is accompanied by their spouse to their NP's office. The LPN documents the following information.

Health History	Nurses' Notes	Vital Signs	Laboratory Results	Healthcare Provider Orders

1430: Client's spouse and children have been noticing increased short-term memory loss in the client over the past 6 months. The client has a history of hypertension and hypothyroidism that are both under control by medication. The client and spouse have been married for 40 years. The client is walking with a cane, which the spouse says the client borrowed from their brother last week without cause. The client's spouse reports that the client has become increasingly irritable and grumpy when the children tell them that they'd forgotten something. They sometimes forget how to use the microwave or the coffee maker. The client states they are hard of hearing and has a lot of trouble sleeping. They tell the LVN they have been "attired" for the past 12 years; the spouse reminds them the word is "retired."

1. NGN Item Type: Matrix Multiple Choice

42.1.1 Use an X for the top six findings that would require immediate follow-up by the nurse.

Patient Findings	Top 6 Findings
Increased short-term memory loss	
Can forget how to use appliances	
History of hypertension	
Newly using a cane without cause	
Uses "attired" instead of "retired"	
Married for 40 years	
Hard of hearing	
Increasingly irritable and grumpy	
Trouble sleeping	

2. NGN Item Type: Multiple Response Select All That Apply

42.1.2 Which nursing assessment findings support the patient's probable diagnosis of Alzheimer's disease? Select all that apply.

A. Older age

B. Hard of hearing

C. Irritable

D. Short-term memory loss

E. Hypertension

      F. Hypothyroidism

      G. Trouble sleeping

      H. Incorrect word usage

      I. Difficulty with familiar task

Scenario

During the visit, the NP discusses common causes of cognitive changes including Alzheimer's disease. Following the visit, the LPN documents in the chart.

Health History	Nurses' Notes	Healthcare Provider Orders	Vital Signs

1500: Reviewed with the client and spouse the options such as medications as presented to them by the NP. A follow-up appointment has been made for 1 month after the tests ordered by the NP to rule out other causes of dementia have been completed.

1. NGN Item Type: Drop-Down Cloze

42.2.1 Choose the *most likely* options for the information missing from the statements below by selecting from the lists of options provided.

Based on the client's current condition, the client's **priority** needs will be to prevent _____1_____, _____2_____, and _____3_____.

Options for 1	Options for 2	Options for 3
Pain	Deep vein thrombosis	Hypertension
Acute confusion	Urinary tract infection	Weight gain
Constipation	Depression	Changes in daily functioning

2. NGN Item Type: Matrix Multiple Response

42.2.2 The LVN is reviewing the plan of care to prevent early complications of Alzheimer's disease. Indicate the appropriate nursing action(s) for each potential complication. Place a number for each nursing action in the appropriate nursing action for each complication; more than one nursing action can be chosen for each complication, each action may only be used once, but not all nursing actions will be used.

Nursing Action	Potential Complications	Appropriate Nursing Action for Each Complication
1. Administer medications as prescribed	Loss of mental abilities	
2. Keep environment free from clutter and safety hazards	Increased confusion	
3. Encourage watching TV or radio during waking hours	Falls	
4. Provide and set a daily routine		
5. Discuss current events		
6. Use restraints for safety		
7. Encourage exercise such as walking		
8. Encourage daily activities such as playing games, painting, or gardening		

Scenario

Two weeks later, the client returns with the spouse and daughter. The NP confirms all other causes of dementia have been ruled out and the final diagnosis is Alzheimer's disease. The family begins to cry, and the client is visibly upset. The NP writes the following order.

Health History	Nurses' Notes	Vital Signs	Laboratory Results	Healthcare Provider Orders

- Donepezil 5 mg po daily at bedtime

1. NGN Item Type: Multiple Response Select N

42.3.1 When reinforcing teaching, the LVN includes which *four* of the following areas?
☐ Take donepezil with food to decrease GI upset.
☐ Watch for increased pulse and blood pressure.
☐ Increase fiber and fluids to decrease constipation.
☐ Choose clothing with buttons to maintain fine motor skills.
☐ Encourage client to continue favorite activities as long as possible.
☐ Other medications can be added as the disease progresses.

Scenario

Eight weeks later, the client and spouse return to the clinic for a follow-up visit. They are more relaxed and able to discuss the treatment plan and progress so far. Following the visit, the LVN documents the following.

Health History	Nurses' Notes	Vital Signs	Laboratory Results

1030: The client reports they have been able to remember their words a little easier. The spouse and children have been referred by the RN to a caregiver's support group. The client reports nausea and some diarrhea daily. They report enjoying golfing with their son-in-law. When the daughter visits, she reports she does everything for her parent to make things easier for them. The client is eating well, and their weight remains stable.

1. NGN Item Type: Highlight Text

42.4.1 Highlight the findings in the nurses' notes that would indicate the client is progressing as expected.

Health History	Nurses' Notes	Vital Signs	Laboratory Results

1030: The client reports they have been able to remember their words a little easier. The spouse and children have been referred by the RN to a caregiver's support group. The client reports nausea and some diarrhea daily. They report enjoying golfing with their son-in-law. When the daughter visits, she reports she does everything for her parent to make things easier for them. The client is eating well, and their weight remains stable.

Constipation

43

Outcome

The student will apply principles of the nursing process and clinical judgment in the care of the client with constipation.

Scenario

The client is a 78-year-old who resides in assisted living in a long-term care (LTC) facility. The practical nurse completes the morning visit, checks the chart, and documents the following:

Health History	Nurses' Notes	Vital Signs	Laboratory Results	Healthcare Provider Orders

The client has a history of a bowel resection for diverticulitis, hypertension diagnosed at age 54, and hypothyroidism for the past 20 years. Medications: levothyroxine, metoprolol, Metamucil, supplements, and vitamins.

Health History	Nurses' Notes	Vital Signs	Laboratory Results	Healthcare Provider Orders

Vital Signs	1000
Temperature (F/C)	97.4°/36.3°
Heart Rate (bpm)	72
Respirations (bpm)	16
Blood Pressure (mmHg)	132/72
Height	5'7"
Weight	188
BMI	29.4

Nurses' Notes

1000:

Subjective: Client states has been lonely since spouse died last year, they used to love to walk together, and "I just don't feel like walking alone." Client likes to take a 20-minute "power nap" every afternoon. Reports still hates the scar on their abdomen from old surgery. Client reports hasn't had much of an appetite lately and feels bloated. Client states just started taking senna and mineral oil. Client says wishes their daughter lived closer so they could see her more often. Client reports painful defecation with dry hard stools with bowel movements every 4 or 5 days. Objective: hypoactive bowel sounds, abdominal distention, abdominal discomfort with palpation in LLQ, labs drawn last week: TSH 3.1 (normal 0.4- 4.0 mU/L)

1. NGN Item Type: Highlight Text

43.1.1 Highlight the client findings that require follow-up by the nurse.

Health History	Nurses' Notes	Vital Signs	Laboratory Results	Healthcare Provider Orders

The client has a history of a bowel resection for diverticulitis, hypertension diagnosed at age 54, and hypothyroidism for the past 20 years. Medications: levothyroxine, metoprolol, Metamucil, supplements, and vitamins.

Health History	Nurses' Notes	Vital Signs	Laboratory Results	Healthcare Provider Orders

Vital Signs	1000
Temperature (F/C)	97.4°/36.3°
Heart Rate (bpm)	72
Respirations (bpm)	16
Blood Pressure (mmHg)	132/72
Height	5'7"
Weight	188
BMI	29.4

Nurses' Notes

1000:

Subjective: Client states has been lonely since spouse died last year, they used to love to walk together, and "I just don't feel like walking alone." Client likes to take a 20-minute "power nap" every afternoon. Reports still hates the scar on their abdomen from old surgery. Client reports hasn't had much of an appetite lately and feels bloated. Client states just started taking senna and mineral oil. Client says wishes their daughter lived closer so they could see her more often. Client reports painful defecation with dry hard stools with bowel movements every 4 or 5 days.

Objective: hypoactive bowel sounds, abdominal distention, abdominal discomfort with palpation in LLQ, labs drawn last week: TSH 3.1

2. NGN Item Type: Drop-Down Cloze

43.1.2 Choose the *most likely* options for the information missing from the statements below by selecting from the lists of options provided.

Based on the client's findings, the practical nursing student determines the findings are consistent with _____1_____ based specifically on _____2_____, _____2_____, and _____2_____.

Options for 1	Options for 2
Bowel obstruction	Takes a power nap
Constipation	BMI 29.4
Encopresis	Painful defecation with dry hard stools
	Doesn't feel like walking
	TSH 3.1
	Hypoactive bowel sounds and abdominal distention
	BM every 4 or 5 days

Scenario

One hour later, the practical nurse has notified the Registered Nurse and the Nurse Practitioner (NP) of their findings and has received new orders.

Health History	Nurses' Notes	Vital Signs	Laboratory Results	Healthcare Provider Orders

1100:

Colace 100 mg po daily

Bisacodyl 10 mg suppository now

Oil retention enema prn

1. NGN Item Type: Multiple Response Select All That Apply

43.2.1 Based on the client's current treatment plan, the client's priority needs will be to prevent which three of the following? Select all that apply.

A. Hemorrhoids

B. Nausea and vomiting

    C. Confusion

    D. Dehydration

    E. Fecal impaction

    F. Reliance on laxatives

    G. Hypertension

    H. Social isolation

2. NGN Item Type: Matrix Multiple Choice

43.2.2 Use an X to indicate which actions listed in the left column would be anticipated by the practical nurse to be included in the plan of care for this patient.

Nursing Actions	Relevant Nursing Actions
Administer stool softeners as ordered	
Administer oral opioids for pain prior to bowel movement	
Encourage total fluid intake of at least 2,500 mL per day	
Assist client in choosing a diet high in fiber	
Ask RN to provide referral to social activities such as a walking group or swimming program	
Document bowel movements with frequency, consistency, and amount	
Reinforce avoiding stimulants such as coffee or tea	
Together with RN, assess for polypharmacy which could contribute to constipation	
Discourage daily "power nap"	
Monitor TSH values for hypothyroidism	

Scenario

The following day, the practical nurse follows up with the client.

Health History	Nurses' Notes	Vital Signs	Laboratory Results	Healthcare Provider Orders

Day 2

1130: Client reports they successfully passed a large, dry stool that morning. States is already feeling less bloated, with less discomfort, and is hungry for lunch. Assessed normoactive bowel sounds. Client asks, "Since I am in assisted living and am on my own, what all can I do to prevent an episode of constipation that bad again?"

1. NGN Item Type: Multiple Response Select N

43.3.1 When reinforcing teaching about constipation, the nurse includes which of the following five statements?

    A. "Some older people think hot water with lemon juice in it upon arising in the morning really helps."

    B. "Continue to get out every day for some exercise like walking or swimming."

    C. "Have some whole-grain bread as toast or with your sandwiches."

    D. "Go ahead and continue taking the senna and mineral oil."

    E. "I've read that prune juice with a carbonated drink can assist with constipation."

    F. "Once you feel you need to have a bowel movement, don't put it off, go take care of it right then."

    G. "Maybe you can call your daughter more often."

    H. "You can cut back on the fluids now that you've passed a stool."

Scenario

The following day, during the practical nurse's daily visit, the client states that they had a smaller but still dry stool that morning. The practical nurse asks the client to tell them what they remember about preventing constipation.

1. NGN Item Type: Matrix Multiple Choice

43.4.1 Use an X to indicate the client statements that indicate successful outcomes.

Client Statement	Successful Outcomes
"I don't need to take my Colace every morning right now while I'm getting over this."	
"I will stop taking the senna and mineral oil, I don't want to have to take that all the time."	
"When I get an urge to go, I'll go to the bathroom right away."	
"My doctor wanted me to get my thyroid levels checked, but I don't need to worry about that now."	
"Raw fruits and veggies are foods I've always liked; I plan on adding more of them to what I eat each day."	
"I will try to eat more white bread and white rice; I like both of those."	
"I went out and got some decaffeinated coffee for me to have from now on."	
"I really enjoy the walking club the RN found for me here, I have been walking every morning."	

44

Dehydration

Outcome

The student will be able to integrate clinical judgment in assessing, planning, implementing, and evaluating care of the client with dehydration.

Scenario

An 80-year-old client has been admitted to the medical unit at the hospital. The practical nurse checks the chart and documents the following findings.

Health History	Nurses' Notes	Healthcare Provider Orders	Laboratory Results

80-year-old client has a history of a hysterectomy at age 57, osteoarthritis, osteoporosis, hypertension, and breast cancer at age 49. Home medications: hydrochlorothiazide 12.5 mg 2 tabs daily, alendronate (Fosamax) weekly, duloxetine (Cymbalta), vitamins, and ibuprofen or acetaminophen as needed for pain.

Health History	Nurses' Notes	Healthcare Provider Orders	Laboratory Results

Vital Signs	1400
Temperature (F/C)	98.6°/37°
Heart Rate (bpm)	110
Respirations (bpm)	18
Blood Pressure (mmHg)	104/60
Height	5'4"
Weight	117 lb
BMI	20.1

Nurses' Notes

1400: Client states is dizzy. Mentation is clear, which daughter reports as baseline. Reports doesn't walk long distances anymore and has stiff, painful knees. Client reports "opening jars is tough" with swollen joints in fingers. Daughter states is worried the client took too many diuretic pills, client's usual weight 125 lb. Client states their "hair has been curly since it grew back after chemotherapy." Decreased skin turgor and dry mucous membrane noted. Urine is dark amber.

Health History	Nurses' Notes	Healthcare Provider Orders	Laboratory Results

Lab Test	Client	Normal
Serum sodium	136 mEq/L	135–145 mEq/L
Urine specific gravity	1.035	1.005–1.025

1. NGN Item Type: Matrix Multiple Choice

44.1.1 Use an X to indicate which client findings require follow-up by the practical nurse at this time.

Client Findings	Assessment Finding That Requires Follow-Up
P 110 and BP 104/60	
R 18	
Client states is dizzy	
Height 5'4'', weight 117, stated usual weight 125	
Decreased skin turgor and dry mucous membranes	
Client states their "hair has been curly since it grew back after chemotherapy"	
Urine is dark amber	
Client states doesn't walk long distances anymore, stiff, painful knees	
Client reports "opening jars is tough" with swollen joints in fingers	
Pertinent labs: Na 155, urine specific gravity 1.035	

2. NGN Item Type: Multiple Response Select All That Apply

44.1.2 Which potential issues may place the client at risk while in the hospital? Select all that apply.
  A. Falls
  B. Orthostatic (postural) hypotension
  C. Confusion
  D. Dependent edema
  E. Hypertension
  F. Weakness and lethargy
  G. ECG changes and cardiac arrhythmias
  H. Nausea and vomiting

Scenario

The practical nurse notes the healthcare provider (HCP) has written orders for the client.

Health History	Nurses' Notes	Healthcare Provider Orders	Laboratory Results

1520:
  - Diagnosis: Dehydration
  - Orthostatic BP
  - Strict I & O
  - VS Q 2 hours
  - Push po fluids
  - D5/0.45% NaCl IV at 75 mL/hr
  - Cardiac monitoring

1. NGN Item Type: Drop-Down Cloze

44.2.1 Choose the *most likely* options for the information missing from the following statements by selecting from the lists of options provided.

Based on the client's current treatment plan, the client's **priority** needs will be to prevent _____1_____ and _____2_____.

Options for 1	Options for 2
Cardiac arrhythmias	Hypertension
Nausea	Weakness
Confusion	Falls

2. NGN Item Type: Matrix Multiple Choice

44.2.2 **Use an X to indicate which actions listed in the left column the practical nurse anticipates would be included in the plan of care for this client.**

Nursing Actions	Implementation
Alert team if cardiac monitor alarms	
Monitor orthostatic BP	
Ask daughter to stay with client around the clock	
Assist RN to closely monitor IV fluids	
Carefully document strict I & O	
Ask for order for restraints to make sure client doesn't fall	
Use "high-risk" fall alert system	
Monitor labs	
If IV fluids fall behind, speed up rate to catch up	
Ask RN to evaluate client for chronic alcohol intake	
Make sure call light is within client's reach	
Routinely assist client to use bedpan or bedside commode	

Scenario

The client has been in hospital for 2 days and is feeling better. The nurse documents most recent information and checks the new lab results. The daughter asks what she can do to "make sure this doesn't happen again."

Health History	Nurses' Notes	Healthcare Provider Orders	Laboratory Results

Day 3

Vital Signs   **1100**

Temperature (F/C)	98.6°/37°
Heart Rate (bpm)	84
Respirations (bpm)	18
Blood Pressure (mmHg)	106/62
Height	5'4"
Weight	115 lb
BMI	20.1

Nurses' Notes

1100: The client shows no confusion, skin turgor is elastic, urine is straw color. Client states they understand how to use their medication box. States knees are still stiff. Discharge orders noted.

Health History	Nurses' Notes	Healthcare Provider Orders	Laboratory Results

Day 3

Lab Test	Client	Normal
Serum sodium	142 mEq/L	135–145 mEq/L
Urine specific gravity	1.015	1.005–1.025

1. NGN Item Type: Matrix Multiple Choice

44.3.1 The practical nurse reinforces teaching for the client and their daughter. Use an X for nursing actions listed below that are <u>indicated</u> (necessary) or <u>contraindicated</u> (could be harmful). Only one selection can be made for each nursing action.

Nursing Action	Indicated	Contraindicated
Get a daily medication box to assist client in administering correct dosage of medications		
Discuss with HCP changing hydrochlorothiazide from 12.5 two tabs once a day to 25 mg once a day		
Ask RN to refer to neuropsychiatrist for Alzheimer's evaluation		
Avoid caffeine and alcohol due to diuretic effects		
Ask RN to refer to home health after discharge to assess home environment		
Reassure daughter this won't happen again		

2. NGN Item Type: Matrix Multiple Choice

44.3.2 For each finding, use an X next to the assessment findings that indicate *successful* outcomes.

Client Findings	Successful Outcomes
BP 106/62	
P 84	
Weight 115	
Skin turgor elastic	
Urine clear straw color	
Urine specific gravity 1.015	
Client states understanding of using medication box	
Client states has stiff, painful knees	

45

End of Life

Outcome

The student will demonstrate comprehensive application of critical thinking in managing the care of the client at the end of life.

Scenario

A 59-year-old client has been placed on home health hospice for terminal ovarian cancer. The LPN is making a first home hospice visit to the client and family.

Health History	Nurses' Notes	Healthcare Provider Orders	Laboratory Results

1130: Client states has put off hospice hoping the last round of chemotherapy would put them in remission, but it did not. Client's son, daughter-in-law, and their two children live in the same town, as does the client's daughter. Client's second daughter and husband and children live out of state. Client states, "The doc told me it could be soon." Client reports is very uncomfortable in the abdomen and around the old surgical site. Client is able to perform their own ADLs. Client is pacing slowly around the room holding on to furniture and is crying and wringing their hands. Client states, "I know I just have to accept this, but I really thought I would recover." Client is visibly upset and trembling and admits to feeling lightheaded this morning. Client states children are not happy with the decision to go on hospice, and they do not want to stress their kids over this. Client has been provided with home oxygen but states they are breathing fine and do not need it.

1. NGN Item Type: Matrix Multiple Choice

45.1.1 Use an X to indicate which patient assessment findings require follow-up by the nurse at this time.

Assessment Finding	Assessment Finding That Requires Follow-Up
Client has put off hospice	
"The doc told me it could be soon"	
Very uncomfortable in their abdomen	
Pacing, crying, wringing their hands	
Is able to perform their own ADLs	
"I know I just have to accept this"	
Client's children are not happy	
Has home oxygen	
Lightheaded	

2. NGN Item Type: Drop-Down Cloze

45.1.2 Choose the *most likely* options for the information missing from the statement below by selecting from the list of options provided.

Based on the client's assessment data, the practice nurse determines the client's _____1_____. _____1_____, _____1_____ may be due to _____2_____ .

Indications for 1	Indications for 2
Crying, pacing, wringing hands	Depression
Upset and trembling	Anxiety
Abdominal pain	Restlessness
Lightheaded	
Able to perform ADLs	
Children are not happy	

Scenario

The client and their family are oriented to hospice care. The following Saturday, the LPN makes a scheduled home visit and a UAP is assisting the client in a partial bed bath.

Health History	Nurses' Notes	Healthcare Provider Orders	Laboratory Results

1345: Client's three children have just arrived and are in the living room together. Client's son states he has been having a difficult time coming to see his parent because it makes him angry. Encouraged the client's children to express their feelings. Client states is in pain more and more, is often unable to sleep, and is worried about being alone. Client states would rather take as few medications as possible so they can visit with their children while they are all here together because they know they won't be able to stay long.

1. NGN Item Type: Multiple Response Select All That Apply

45.2.1 Based on the patient's current treatment plan, the patient's priority needs will be to prevent which of the following? Select all that apply.
A. Confusion
B. Pain
C. Addiction
D. Anger
E. Hope
F. Loneliness

2. NGN Item Type: Multiple Response Select N

45.2.2 Select the six items that the LPN will include when reinforcing teaching to the client and family.
☐ Importance of adequate pain control
☐ What to expect as death nears
☐ Options for assisted suicide
☐ Value of meeting any religious and cultural needs
☐ Hospice staff will work to assist client and family to make end of life comfortable
☐ Progressing through the states of the grieving process
☐ Stressed importance of IV hydration
☐ Client is in control of their own decisions in experiencing a good death

Scenario

Ten days later, the LPN is now making brief daily visits and documents their findings.

Health History	Nurses' Notes	Healthcare Provider Orders	Laboratory Results

0930: On arrival, client was in bed with their children and their families at the bedside. Client is in visible pain and moaning. Client states has not urinated today and has not had a bowel movement in 5 days. Respirations are 11, shallow, and noisy. Client's daughter states, "Please do something!" Notified hospice NP and received new orders.

Health History	Nurses' Notes	Healthcare Provider Orders	Laboratory Results

Around-the-clock slow-release oral morphine
Sublingual morphine prn for breakthrough pain

1. NGN Item Type: Matrix Multiple Choice

45.3.1 Use an X for nursing actions listed below that are <u>indicated</u> (necessary), <u>contraindicated</u> (could be harmful), or <u>nonessential</u> (not necessary). Only one selection can be made for each nursing action.

Nursing Action	Indicated	Contraindicated	Nonessential
Teach family how to give foot and backrubs			
Set up pain analgesia around-the-clock schedule per NP orders			
Encourage family and client to follow religious or cultural practices			
Remind client not to ask for too much prn pain medication to not become addicted			
Reinforce teaching regarding how morphine will assist with breathing, pain, and anxiety			
Push the client to take fluids orally			
Open the bedroom curtains to let in light			
Encourage the client to remain in bed			
Make sure there are fresh flowers in the room			

Scenario

Two days later, the nurse makes a visit after a call from the hospice home health UAP.

Health History	Nurses' Notes	Healthcare Provider Orders	Laboratory Results

0715: Client's daughter states that mom is sleeping more and more. Hospice home health UAP states client has not eaten anything since the day before yesterday and has had nothing to drink for over 24 hours. Client is groaning in pain and is moving restlessly. Client's pulse is 48, weak and thready, respirations 8 and irregular, and blood pressure is obtained by palpation at 86/42. Client has a stage 2 pressure injury on bilateral heels. Family is at the bedside together, telling favorite stories together. Client whispers, "It's OK, it's OK, I love you all, it's going to be OK," and wants to hug each family member.

1. NGN Item Type: Highlight Text

45.4.1 **Highlight the findings that indicate the patient is transitioning as expected in end-of-life care.**

| Health History | Nurses' Notes | Healthcare Provider Orders | Laboratory Results |

0715: Client's daughter states that mom is sleeping more and more. Hospice home health UAP states client has not eaten anything since the day before yesterday and has had nothing to drink for over 24 hours. Client is groaning in pain and is moving restlessly. Client's pulse is 48, weak and thready, respirations 8 and irregular, and blood pressure is obtained by palpation at 86/42. Client has a stage 2 pressure injury on bilateral heels. Family is at the bedside together, telling favorite stories together. Client whispers, "It's OK, it's OK, I love you all, it's going to be OK," and wants to hug each family member.

46

Falls

Outcome

The student will use clinical judgment in nursing management of a patient with an increased risk for falls.

Scenario

The client is 76 years old and lives in a little house alone just across the street from their daughter. The practical nurse working in the Emergency Department documents the following findings.

Health History	Nurses' Notes	Healthcare Provider Orders	Laboratory Results

Daughter called 911 when she found 76-year-old client had fallen at home. Admitted to emergency department. Client has stage 1 heart failure and well-controlled diabetes mellitus type 2. Client's current medications include hydrochlorothiazide and metformin.

Health History	Nurses' Notes	Healthcare Provider Orders	Laboratory Results

Vital Signs	0845
Temperature (F/C)	97.6°/36.4°
Heart Rate (bpm)	90
Respirations (bpm)	18
Blood Pressure (mmHg)	132/74

Nurses' Notes

0845: Daughter states client has fallen several times in the past few months, but this time the daughter was unable to get the client up from the floor. Client reports poor balance and states doesn't feel any injuries "other than to my pride." Client's daughter reports client holds on to furniture when walking around house as much as possible. Client has worn glasses for the past 22 years. Client reports occasional pins and needles and numbness in feet and urinary frequency in the evening. Noted 1+ edema bilateral ankles, lungs clear to auscultation, fingerstick blood sugar 105 at arrival to ED.

1. NGN Item Type: Matrix Multiple Choice Select N

46.1.1 Use an X for the top *four* findings that would require immediate follow-up to the box on the right.

Client Findings	Top 4 Findings
VS: T 97.6°F (36.4°C), P 90, R 18, BP 132/74	
Client reports poor balance	
Client's daughter reports client holds on to furniture as much as possible	
Client has worn glasses for the past 22 years	
1+ edema bilateral ankles	
Lungs clear to auscultation	
Client reports occasional pins and needles and numbness in feet	
Blood sugar 105	
Client reports urinary frequency in the evening	
Client states doesn't feel any injuries "other than to my pride"	

2. NGN Item Type: Drag-and-Drop Cloze

46.1.2 Based on the assessment findings, choose the *most likely* options for the information missing from the statements below by selecting from the lists of options provided.

The practical nurse determines the client's falls are most likely due to _____1_____ and _____2_____.

Options for 1	Options for 2
Vision	Heart failure
Diabetes	Hydrochlorothiazide
Neuropathy	Metformin

Scenario

Several hours later, while settling the client into bed, the daughter tells the practical nurse that the client has always liked taking their medications right before dinner. After reviewing the Healthcare Provider Orders, the practical nurse works with the RN in planning care for the client.

Health History	Nurses' Notes	Healthcare Provider Orders	Laboratory Results

Admit to observation unit for overnight stay
Anticipated discharge tomorrow

1. NGN Item Type: Multiple Response Select All That Apply

46.2.1 Based on the patient's current condition, the client's priority needs will be to prevent which of the following? Select all that apply.
- A. Client injury
- B. Stress ulcer
- C. Confusion
- D. Further falls
- E. Altered nutrition
- F. Constipation
- G. Loneliness
- H. Fractures (i.e., hip)

2. NGN Item Type: Matrix Multiple Choice

46.2.2 Use an X for the nursing actions listed below that are <u>indicated</u> (appropriate or necessary) or <u>contraindicated</u> (could be harmful) for the client's care at this time. Only one selection can be made for each nursing action.

Nursing Action	Indicated	Contraindicated
Tell the patient to stay in bed		
Reinforce teaching to take daily medications in the morning		
Prepare to administer oral antibiotic		
Make sure call light is within reach, and answer it promptly		
Assist RN with fear of falling assessment		
Prepare client to go to long-term care center		
Remind the client to decrease oral fluid intake		
Assist RN to complete a thorough assessment of client's feet		
Turn every 2 hours		
Reinforce teaching regarding use of a cane to stabilize gait		

Scenario

The client is discharged home, and 2 days later, a home health LPN makes a home visit. The daughter is present for the visit. After reinforcing teaching, the nurse documents the client's response.

Health History	Nurses' Notes	Healthcare Provider Orders	Laboratory Results

1445: Reinforced safety teaching to the daughter and client. The client states, "The grab bars for the bathroom will be installed this weekend and my son-in-law installed a raised toilet seat." Daughter reports the loose rugs around the house have been removed. Client states, "I really don't like the cane they gave me, it's ugly so I don't use it." Client reports already switched over the hydrochlorothiazide to take it just in the morning and states, "I don't really need my glasses that much and I forget to wear them anyway, and it's probably fine." Daughter states, "We found a cute nightlight for the bathroom, and one for the hallway."

---

1. NGN Item Type: Matrix Multiple Choice

46.3.1 Use an X to indicate which actions listed in the left column the practical nurse would include in reinforcing teaching with this client.

Nursing Actions	Implemented
Floors can be slippery, so make sure you are wearing slippers or nonskid socks.	
Do passive range of motion exercises daily.	
Monitor your vital signs at home at least three times a day.	
Make sure you have your rooms well lit so that you can see well.	
Your daughter will provide all your care necessary, so you don't need to worry.	
Reinforce how to use home oxygen.	
Handrails in the bathroom would be a really good idea to have installed.	
Make sure to wear your glasses, you may want to get a chain around your neck so you can find them.	
Pay special attention to uneven surfaces or stairs.	

---

2. NGN Item Type: Matrix Multiple Choice

46.3.2 Use an X next to the client statements that indicate successful outcomes.

Patient Statement	Successful Outcomes
"The grab bars for the bathroom will be installed this weekend."	
"I really don't like the cane they gave me, it's ugly so I don't use it."	
"My daughter removed the loose rugs I have out."	
"I've already switched over the hydrochlorothiazide to take it just in the morning."	
"I don't really need my glasses that much and I forget to wear them anyway, and it's probably fine."	
"My son-in-law installed a raised toilet seat."	
"We found a cute nightlight for the bathroom, and one for the hallway."	

Outcome

The student will prioritize the key aspects of nursing management of the client with urinary incontinence.

Scenario

An 82-year-old client has been admitted to a long-term care center for rehabilitation. The practical nurse enters the room at the beginning of the shift and notices a strong urine odor and wet linens. The nurse documents the following findings.

Health History	Nurses' Notes	Vital Signs	Laboratory Results

82-year-old client admitted following a stroke, client was transferred from hospital where they spent 3 weeks recovering. Client was diagnosed with benign prostatic hypertrophy while in hospital.

Health History	Nurses' Notes	Healthcare Provider Orders	Laboratory Results

Vital Signs	1130
Temperature (F/C)	97.8°/36.5°
Heart Rate (bpm)	72
Respirations (bpm)	16
Blood Pressure (mmHg)	126/72

Nurses' Notes

1130 Assessment:

Subjective
- Client states, "I'm so embarrassed about the smell, I'm not sure what's happening."
- Speech slightly slurred but spouse states it is "so much better"

Objective
- Right hand grip 4/5
- Left hand grip 5/5
- Minimal bilateral leg weakness
- Slightly unsteady when ambulating
- Client incontinent of urine

1. NGN Item Type: Drop-Down Cloze

47.1.1 Choose the *most likely* options for the information missing from the statements below by selecting from the lists of options provided.

The client findings that require immediate follow-up include _____1_____, _____2_____, _____3_____.

Options for 1	Options for 2	Options for 3
Left hand grip 5/5	Wet linens	BP 126/72
Strong urine odor	Slightly unsteady when ambulating	Speech slightly slurred
Minimal bilateral leg weakness	T 97.8°F (36.5°C)	"I'm so embarrassed by the smell"

2. NGN Item Type: Matrix Multiple Choice

47.1.2 Use an X to indicate which potential issues listed in the left column may place this client at risk while in the long-term care center.

Potential Issue	Risk to Patient
Falls	
Skin breakdown	
Venous thrombus emboli	
Constipation	
Bladder cancer	
Body image disturbance	

Scenario

An ordered urine culture and sensitivity were sent, and the following day the results returned as negative for infection. The practical nurse and the charge nurse work on a plan of care for the client.

Health History	Nurses' Notes	Healthcare Provider Orders	Laboratory Results

Day 2

Nurses' Notes

0830: Bladder palpated, distended, and tender. Bladder scan shows residual urine 300 mL. Client states that this never happened before the stroke and states, "I don't always feel the need to pee."

1. NGN Item Type: Multiple Response Select All That Apply

47.2.1 The practical nurse will ask which priority questions to gather additional information about the patient's highest priority needs? Select all that apply.

A. "When did the urine leakage start?"

B. Have you ever had an indwelling catheter?"

C. "Have you noticed if the leaks occur more in the daytime or at night?"

D. "Are you having trouble going to the bathroom or using the urinal on time?"

E. "Are you allergic to contrast media?"

2. NGN Item Type: Matrix Multiple Choice

47.2.2 Use an X to indicate which actions listed in the left column would be anticipated in the plan of care for this patient.

Nursing Actions	Anticipated in Plan of Care
Inspect and monitor the skin	
Prepare to insert an indwelling catheter	
Remind client to call for assistance when needing to urinate	
Collaborate with the Registered Nurse to assess for functional ability to manipulate clothing for toileting	
Decrease oral intake of fluids	
Assess for signs of overhydration, such as crackles in the lungs and pedal edema	

Scenario

The following day, the rehabilitation team has met to plan a bladder training program for the client. Following the meeting, the nurse checks the chart for new orders and documents findings.

Health History	Nurses' Notes	**Healthcare Provider Orders**	Laboratory Results

Postvoid residual bladder scan
Tamsulosin 0.4 mg orally once daily

Health History	**Nurses' Notes**	Healthcare Provider Orders	Laboratory Results

Day 3
Nurses' Notes
1530: Repeat bladder scan postvoid residual urine 280 mL. Client reports feels has been "dribbling pee a lot."

1. NGN Item Type: Matrix Multiple Choice

47.3.1 Use an X to indicate which actions listed in the left column would be included in the plan of care for this patient.

Nursing Actions	Implementation
Discuss the possibility with the RN of using a condom catheter at night	
Reinforce teaching on Kegel exercises	
Instruct the nursing assistant about a toileting schedule	
Administer tamsulosin (Flomax) as prescribed	
Remind client it is expected that they will remain free of incontinence	
Inspect the skin with each incontinence episode for incontinence-associated dermatitis	
Remind patient to go to the toilet every 4 hours	
Prepare to collect a 24-hour urine sample	
Provide clothing with Velcro for ease of access	
Teach client to double void to fully empty bladder	

Scenario

The practical nurse comes on duty after being off for a week and reassesses the client's progress.

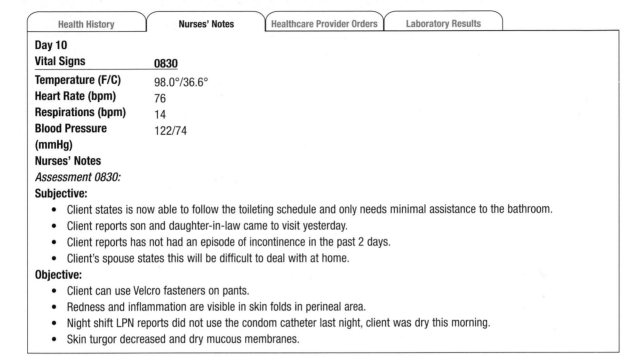

Health History	Nurses' Notes	Healthcare Provider Orders	Laboratory Results

Day 10

Vital Signs	0830
Temperature (F/C)	98.0°/36.6°
Heart Rate (bpm)	76
Respirations (bpm)	14
Blood Pressure (mmHg)	122/74

Nurses' Notes

Assessment 0830:

Subjective:

- Client states is now able to follow the toileting schedule and only needs minimal assistance to the bathroom.
- Client reports son and daughter-in-law came to visit yesterday.
- Client reports has not had an episode of incontinence in the past 2 days.
- Client's spouse states this will be difficult to deal with at home.

Objective:

- Client can use Velcro fasteners on pants.
- Redness and inflammation are visible in skin folds in perineal area.
- Night shift LPN reports did not use the condom catheter last night, client was dry this morning.
- Skin turgor decreased and dry mucous membranes.

---

1. NGN Item Type: Matrix Multiple Choice

47.4.1 For each assessment finding, use an X to indicate whether the interventions were <u>effective</u> (helped to meet expected outcomes), <u>ineffective</u> (did not help to meet expected outcomes), or <u>unrelated</u> (not related to the expected outcomes).

Assessment Finding	Effective	Ineffective	Unrelated
Client can use Velcro fasteners on pants			
Client reports has not had an episode of incontinence in the past 2 days			
Redness and inflammation are visible in skin folds in perineal area			
Client reports son and daughter-in-law came to visit yesterday			
Night shift LPN reports did not use the condom catheter last night, client was dry this morning			
VS: T 98.0°F (36.6°C), P 76, R 14, BP 122/74			
Client's spouse states this will be difficult to deal with at home			
Skin turgor decreased and dry mucous membranes			
Client states is now able to follow the toileting schedule and only needs minimal assistance to the bathroom			

48 Wound Care

Outcome

The student will demonstrate comprehensive application of critical thinking in managing the care of the client with complex wound care needs.

Scenario

A 72-year-old client is sent from a clinic as a direct admission to their local hospital's medical floor. The nurse reviews the client's history and documents the admission vital signs in the nurses' notes.

Health History	Nurses' Notes	Healthcare Provider Orders	Laboratory Results

Client is 72 years old with history of diabetes mellitus type 2 and hypertension. Client sent from a clinic as a direct admission for a left foot wound that is not healing. Client lives at home with spouse and states, "We had a trip planned to see our son and his family in a few weeks." Client states that they have been taking care of the wound at home for a week and changed the bandage on the left foot yesterday. Client states the wound looked a little red all the way around it and went to the clinic where they assessed and redressed the wound. Client is on a vegetarian diet, tries to watch sweets intake, and smoked years ago in college. Client states, "This is awful. I love to be outside. Today I had to miss a golf game." Client's current medications include metformin, lisinopril, and multiple vitamins and has been taking either Tylenol 1000 mg or hydrocodone/acetaminophen 5/25, but began alternating with ibuprofen because has not had a good bowel movement for days.

Health History	Nurses' Notes	Healthcare Provider Orders	Laboratory Results

Vital Signs	1300
Temperature (F/C)	99.2°/37.3°
Heart Rate (bpm)	82
Respirations (bpm)	16
Blood Pressure (mmHg)	126/72
Height	5'11"
Weight	223 lb
BMI	31.1

---

1. NGN Item Type: Multiple Response Select All That Apply

48.1.1 Which of the following client assessment findings require immediate follow-up? Select all that apply.

- A. History of diabetes mellitus type 2
- B. Left foot wound that is not healing
- C. Taking care of the wound at home for a week
- D. Changed the bandage on left foot yesterday
- E. The wound looked a little red all the way around it
- F. Vegetarian diet
- G. Smoked years ago in college
- H. T 99.8°F (37.6°C)
- I. Ht 5'11", Wt 223, BMI 31.1
- J. No bowel movement

2. NGN Item Type: Drop-Down Cloze

48.1.2 Choose the *most likely* **options for the information missing from the statement below by selecting from the list of options provided.**

The nurse recognizes that, based on the client's history, the client is currently at risk for complications, including _____1_____, _____2_____, and _____3_____.

Indications for 1	Indications for 2	Indications for 3
Thrombophlebitis	Cellulitis	Keloid scarring
Pneumonia	Wound evisceration	Constipation
Wound infection	Shock	Adhesions

Scenario

The practical nurse settles the client in the room, assesses the client, documents the findings, and then checks the lab results in the client's chart.

Health History	Nurses' Notes	Healthcare Provider Orders	Laboratory Results

Nurses' Notes

1500:

- Alert and oriented × 3
- S1S2 noted, no chest pain reported
- Lungs are clear to auscultation, no SOB or cough
- Abdomen soft and nontender, reports usual bowel movement daily, last one yesterday
- Voids without difficulty
- Skin warm, dry, and intact
- Left foot dressing clean, dry, and intact
- Pain currently 6/10 (0–10 scale)

Health History	Nurses' Notes	Healthcare Provider Orders	Laboratory Results

Lab Test	Client	Normal
Serum potassium	4.7 mEq/L	3.5–5.0 mEq/L
Albumin	3.1 g/dL	3.3–5.2 g/dL
HgbA1c	6.7%	4–5.6%
Serum glucose	132 mg/dL	70–100 mg/dL
White blood cell count	10,580 mm³	4,500–11,000 mm³

1. NGN Item Type: Drop-Down Cloze

48.2.1 Choose the *most likely* **options for the information missing from the statements below by selecting from the lists of options provided.**

Based on the client's current treatment plan, the client's **priority** need will be _____1_____ as evidenced by the client's _____2_____, _____2_____, and _____2_____.

Options for 1	Options for 2
Constipation	Delayed healing
Wound evisceration	Home wound care for a week
Wound care	Fistula formation
	Abdominal wound
	Potential wound infection

2. NGN Item Type: Multiple Response Grouping

48.2.2 Based on the client findings, select the anticipated HCP orders from each of the following categories. (Each category must have at least one response option selected.)

Category	Orders
Imaging	☐ Chest x-ray
	☐ X-ray left foot
	☐ Ultrasound left foot
Medications	☐ Hydrocodone/acetaminophen 5/325 mg 1 po Q 4–6 hrs prn pain
	☐ Ducosate 100 mg 1 po daily
	☐ Prednisone 20 mg one po Q am
Interventions	☐ Low-protein diet
	☐ Wound irrigation followed by packing wound and wet-to-dry dressing changed daily
	☐ Montgomery straps to secure dressing
	☐ Transparent film dressing, change Q 3 days
	☐ Obtain wound culture

Scenario

Three days later, the client is anticipating discharge home.

Health History	**Nurses' Notes**	Healthcare Provider Orders	Laboratory Results

Day 4

Vital Signs	**1000**
Temperature (F/C)	98.4°/36.8°
Heart Rate (bpm)	72
Respirations (bpm)	16
Blood Pressure (mmHg)	128/76

Nurses' Notes

1000: Client anticipating discharge home. RN has scheduled home health visits twice a week. Client will change left foot dressing dressing on the days the home health LPN is not there. Dietician has seen client to discuss nutritional needs for wound healing and lowering the hemoglobin A1c. Teaching reinforced and effectiveness of care evaluated.

Health History	Nurses' Notes	Healthcare Provider Orders	**Laboratory Results**

Day 4

Lab Test	Client	Normal
White blood cell count	9,211 mm^3	4,500–11, 000 mm^3

1. NGN Item Type: Matrix Multiple Choice

48.3.1 Use an X for the nursing actions listed below that are <u>indicated</u> (appropriate or necessary) or <u>contraindicated</u> (could be harmful) for the client's care at this time. Only one selection can be made for each nursing action.

Nursing Action	Indicated	Contraindicated
"Let's go over these supplies I am sending home with you for your first dressing change tomorrow."		
Reinforce signs and symptoms of wound infection to report		
"Keeping your blood sugar within the prescribed range is very important."		
Discuss the value of good nutrition in wound healing		
Reinforce steps to remove the sutures		
Reinforce the steps in proper handwashing for dressing changes		
Provide written instructions for wound care and dressing changes		
Reinforce the use of Montgomery straps		
Remind the client not to get the dressing wet		

2. NGN Item Type: Extended Multiple Response Select All That Apply

48.3.2 Which of the following findings indicate effectiveness? Select all that apply.
   A. The wound is clean and dry without redness or swelling.
   B. The wound drainage is sanguineous.
   C. Client reports pain 2/10 on 0 to 10 scale.
   D. Return demonstration of dressing change properly performed by client.
   E. The client states they will increase carbohydrates and decrease protein.
   F. The culture was negative for infection.

Outcome

The student will use clinical judgment in nursing management utilizing therapeutic communication.

Scenario

A 58-year-old client has been assigned to a home health LPN. The LPN is getting ready to make the first visit together with a nursing student. Prior to the visit, the LPN and the student review the client's chart, medications, and history. The LPN asks the student to tell them what they know about therapeutic communication.

Health History	Nurses' Notes	Vital Signs	Laboratory Results

58-year-old client with history of cancer, depression, and anxiety. Recently discharged from the hospital for a mental health inpatient visit.

1. NGN Item Type: Multiple Response Select N

49.1.1   Use an X to indicate the *three* student statements that would require follow-up by the LPN.

Student Statements	Three Student Statements Requiring Follow-Up
"Verbal communication is anything spoken, is in writing, or uses language or symbols."	
"Therapeutic communication focuses on giving treatment."	
"Communication uses both listening and interacting."	
"Nonverbal communication is done without speaking; it is using body language or motions."	
"I need to make sure what I say matches my nonverbal messages."	
"I want to get good at communicating and then I can use the same style with everyone."	
"I will use intrapersonal communication when I talk with the client."	

2. NGN Item Type: Multiple Response Select N

49.1.2   Which of the following *four* statements place the student at risk for nontherapeutic communication?

A. "I like to ask personal questions to help the client feel relaxed."
B. "It helps me to repeat what the client has said in my own words."
C. "I have a good sense of humor that can help when it is appropriate to do so."
D. "Sometimes it is OK to change the subject if it gets too uncomfortable."
E. "I like to ask a lot of why questions that help to explain why the person is acting that way."
F. "Sometimes the best thing for me to do is say nothing, and just be quiet."
G. "Saying things like 'I'm so sorry' lets the client know that I care."

Scenario

After the visit with the client, the LPN and the nursing student return to the home health office. They sit down to discuss nontherapeutic communication and what they anticipate will be included in the plan of care to establish communication that is centered on the client's needs.

1. NGN Item Type: Drop-Down Cloze

49.2.1 Choose the *most likely* options for the information missing from the student nurse's statement below by selecting from the list of options provided.

"Nontherapeutic communication is a _____1_____ between the nurse and the client in establishing a trusting helpful relationship. When the nurse does not use therapeutic communication, it can _____2_____ communication and can stop the client from reaching their treatment goals. Incongruent communication can be easy to do as a nurse if I am tired or distracted and my verbal and nonverbal messages don't _____3_____. I need to remember that every interaction matters."

Options for 1	Options for 2	Options for 3
option	block	reassure
barrier	encourage	match
summary	focus	educate

2. NGN Item Type: Matrix Multiple Choice

49.2.2 Use an X to indicate which actions listed in the left column would be included in the plan of care to develop therapeutic communication with this client.

Nursing Actions	Implementation
Verify understanding directly by stating, "Do you understand me?"	
Use mindfulness to listen to what the client is saying without being distracted.	
Assess the client's nonverbal communication such as posture and hand movements.	
Ask yes or no questions to gather specific information.	
Do not interrupt, allow the client to finish speaking.	
Assess the client's readiness to communicate.	
Clarify anything the client said that you are not sure you understood.	
Encourage eye contact and use therapeutic touch.	

Scenario

The client who was scheduled after lunch cancels their appointment. The LPN and the student nurse use the time to practice therapeutic communication. The LPN gives the student practice client statements and assists the student to analyze the responses.

1. NGN Item Type: Matrix Multiple Choice

49.3.1 Use an X to indicate which nursing student responses listed in the left column are therapeutic or nontherapeutic responses. Only one selection can be made for each nursing student response.

Nursing Student Response	Therapeutic	Nontherapeutic
"If I were you, I would definitely go and see that doctor."		
"I'm not sure I understood that, can you tell me more?"		
"Don't worry, everything will be OK, I'm sure of it."		
"Why are you so upset?"		
"You shouldn't even think about that, it's just not right."		
"I need you to lower your voice when you're speaking to me."		
"I'm impressed with how well you are handling the stress of your move."		
"You know that isn't true."		
"What is one thing you could do to feel better right now?"		

Scenario

At the end of the clinical day, the LPN and nursing student review therapeutic communication and what has been discussed and practiced.

1. NGN Item Type: Multiple Response Select All That Apply

49.4.1 Which of the following nursing student statements indicate successful learning outcomes? Select all that apply.

A. "A respectful and caring style of communication can assist in developing a therapeutic relationship."

B. "It takes time, patience, and practice to develop therapeutic communication techniques."

C. "The client who refuses to communicate should be left alone."

D. "Therapeutic listening is a key component to therapeutic communication."

E. "It is important to adapt to the client's preferred cultural style of communication."

F. "Letting go of personal stress and providing a calm environment can assist in effective communication."

Delegation

Outcome

The student will demonstrate comprehensive application of critical thinking in using the skills of delegation.

Scenario

A.B. is a 26-year-old nursing student assigned to a leadership clinical rotation. A.B. is working with a nurse who has been an LVN for 16 years. They are working on a 28-bed medical-surgical floor. Staffing today consists of an RN charge nurse, two RN staff nurses each with four clients, two LVNs each with six clients, and two unlicensed assistive personnel (UAP). The LVN working with A.B. has been assigned the following six clients.

Client 1	81-year-old client with asthma exacerbation, history of asthma, dementia, and breast cancer, currently short of breath, dyspneic, oxygen saturation 89%
Client 2	49-year-old client who had surgery 2 days ago for knee replacement, history of severe osteoarthritis in bilateral knees, continues to have issues with pain control, due for discharge tomorrow
Client 3	68-year-old client with longstanding history of diabetes mellitus type 2 with diabetic ketoacidosis on an insulin drip and aggressive IV fluid and electrolyte replacement with frequent blood sugar monitoring
Client 4	64-year-old client with suspected abdominal blockage, history of abdominal adhesions following a colectomy, currently is NPO
Client 5	78-year-old client transferred yesterday from long-term care with exacerbation of diverticular disease and ileostomy, currently the ileostomy is leaking around the stoma
Client 6	56-year-old new admission with suspected sepsis following outpatient oral surgery, client's blood pressure is dropping and is now hypotensive

1. NGN Item Type: Highlight Table

50.1.1 Highlight the findings for each client that requires follow-up by the LVN.

Client 1	81-year-old client with asthma exacerbation, history of asthma, dementia, and breast cancer, currently short of breath, dyspneic, oxygen saturation 89%
Client 2	49-year-old client who had surgery 2 days ago for knee replacement, history of severe osteoarthritis in bilateral knees, continues to have issues with pain control, due for discharge tomorrow
Client 3	68-year-old client with longstanding history of diabetes mellitus type 2 with diabetic ketoacidosis on an insulin drip and aggressive IV fluid and electrolyte replacement with frequent blood sugar monitoring
Client 4	64-year-old client with suspected abdominal blockage, history of abdominal adhesions following a colectomy, currently is NPO
Client 5	78-year-old client transferred yesterday from long-term care with exacerbation of diverticular disease and ileostomy, currently the ileostomy is leaking around the stoma
Client 6	56-year-old new admission with suspected sepsis following outpatient oral surgery, client's blood pressure is dropping and is now hypotensive

2. NGN Item Type: Multiple Response Select N

50.1.2 Use an X to indicate which two clients the student nurse should question as inappropriate to the LVN's assignment.

Clients	Inappropriate Assignment
81-year-old client with asthma exacerbation, history of asthma, dementia, and breast cancer, currently short of breath, dyspneic, oxygen saturation 89%	
49-year-old client who had surgery 2 days ago for knee replacement, history of severe osteoarthritis in bilateral knees, continues to have issues with pain control, due for discharge tomorrow	
68-year-old client with longstanding history of diabetes mellitus type 2 with diabetic ketoacidosis on an insulin drip and aggressive IV fluid and electrolyte replacement with frequent blood sugar monitoring	
64-year-old client with suspected abdominal blockage, history of abdominal adhesions following a colectomy, currently is NPO	
78-year-old client transferred yesterday from long-term care with exacerbation of diverticular disease and ileostomy, currently the ileostomy is leaking around the stoma	
56-year-old new admission with suspected sepsis following outpatient oral surgery, client's blood pressure is dropping and is now hypotensive	

Scenario

The LVN approaches the charge nurse with concerns about the assigned clients. Due to the high acuity of the clients on the unit today, the charge nurse states that reassigning clients will not be possible. The charge nurse tells the LVN that they or one of the other RNs will assist with anything outside of the LVN's scope of practice and education.

1. NGN Item Type: Drop-Down Cloze

50.2.1 The LVN and student nurse A.B. discuss assignment and delegation. The LVN asks A.B. to state what they remember about delegation. Choose the *most likely options* for the missing information below.

"I need to first know my state and facility's _____1_____ so I know what I can and cannot do. If I delegate a selected duty, I have transferred _____2_____, and so I must delegate carefully. The LVN is _____3_____ for anything that is delegated. Any work that is delegated must be given to a person that is _____4_____ in that task or skill."

Options for 1 and 2	Options for 3 and 4
Authority	Legal
Supervision	Competent
Confidence	Appropriate
Scope of practice	Accountable
Safety	Monitoring

2. NGN Item Type: Matrix Multiple Choice

50.2.2 The LVN and A.B. plan their care for their shift. Use an X to identify which interventions can be performed by the LVN and which will need to be completed only by the RN. Only one choice can be made per intervention.

Nursing Interventions	LVN	RN
Calculate and titrate an IV dopamine drip to blood pressure		
Administer oral antibiotics		
Place an NG tube		
Develop the full plan of care for the new admission		
Change the ileostomy appliance		
Change the oxygen setting to raise oxygen saturation		
Administer oral pain medications		

Scenario

After lunch, A.B. makes up a list of the afternoon activities and tasks to be accomplished. The LVN and A.B. review the list together.

1. NGN Item Type: Multiple Response Select N

50.3.1 Which *five* of the following tasks and activities would be appropriate for the nurse to delegate to the UAP?
   A. Inserting an indwelling urinary catheter
   B. Make up the surgical bed
   C. Provide oral hygiene
   D. Adjust the oxygen level on the nasal cannula
   E. Assist client to the bedside commode
   F. Reinforce teaching about insulin
   G. Enter intake and output in the computer
   H. Assess the client's pain level
   I. Transferring the client to the chair at the bedside

2. NGN Item Type: Matrix Multiple Choice

50.3.2 At the end of the student's clinical shift, the LVN assesses the student's learning. Use an X next to the student statements that indicate successful outcomes.

Student Statement	Successful Outcomes
"When I get a job, I'll carefully review the agency policies on what the UAP can and cannot do."	
"I can delegate the things I don't really like to do."	
"The RN must complete most of the steps of the nursing process."	
"I'll never forget to check my own client assignment to make sure it is appropriate."	
"It is OK if I delegate vital signs to the UAP on clients who are not physiologically stable."	